Kathleen

Thanks for your interest
on my work

regards,

DR. Pereira

Begin in March... Out of hell does he come

Only then does the Lost shepherd

To the armies of the Lamb return to do battle

With olive wreath that rests upon head

Sitting in Lotus, staff in hand that brakes then heals

The heart torn from the rib of Adam...

When He who cannot be found but does only rest

Begins the ascent upon White Swan.

Then does a Brahma awaken...

From out of a navel of an Ocean of Consciousness...

That, which began and is again and again...

Always, pulsing through its Crown

First through the ether

Vibrating throughout the astral realms

What first begins as darkness in a karmic field...

Can then verily become Light to its Brachman.

— Robert B. Pereira

Faces of
Dual Diagnosis

A Canadian Perspective

Robert B. Pereira, MD

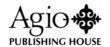

Agio
PUBLISHING HOUSE

PUBLISHING HOUSE

151 Howe Street, Victoria BC Canada V8V 4K5

The author of this book does not advocate the use of any technique
as form of treatment for physical or medical problems without the
advice of a physician, either directly or indirectly. The intent of the
author is only to offer information of a general nature to help you
in your quest for physical fitness and good mental and spiritual
health. In the event you use any of the information in this book for
yourself, which is your right, the author and the publisher assume
no responsibility for your actions.

*For rights information and bulk orders,
please contact:*
info@agiopublishing.com
or go to
www.agiopublishing.com

Faces of Dual Diagnosis
ISBN 978-1-897435-52-6 (laminated hardcover)

For more information, we invite you to visit
www.DualDiagnosis.ca

Printed on acid-free paper that includes no fibre
from endangered forests. Agio Publishing House is a
socially responsible company, measuring success on
a triple-bottom-line basis.

10 9 8 7 6 5 4 3 2 1 0

DEDICATION

This manuscript is dedicated to the memory of my parents:
Philip Pereira, who taught me the importance of virtue, and
Marlene Pereira, who gave me a practical understanding of faith.

ACKNOWLEDGMENTS

I first wish to thank my patients, who have taught me so much over the years, and in particular, the individuals portrayed in the case studies within for sharing their stories.

I wish to acknowledge Dr. Gabor Maté, whose courage and tenacity have been an inspiration to me both personally and professionally, and Dr. Karima Jiwa, my mentor, whose patience and understanding have provided an environment to grow and realize my potential.

I also wish to acknowledge my editor, Diana Holland, who has worked tirelessly with me toward the realization of a dream.

I wish to thank Bruce and Marsha Batchelor at Agio Publishing House for enabling this labor to come to fruition.

Finally, I wish to thank my wife, Lucia Maria, without whose love and support my career and life would not have flourished.

TABLE OF CONTENTS

AUTHOR'S NOTE

My interest in writing this book stems from my professional experience in dealing with dually diagnosed individuals for almost two decades. Some of my patients have managed to springboard themselves into a life of stability and relative contentment. Others, sadly, devolved sooner or later toward a hopeless condition of both body and mind.

What has increasingly captivated my interest has been the role of belief systems in those who have braved the gauntlet and won. I have discovered that in almost every case, a conscious decision on the part of the individual *not* to personalize his or her experiences opened the door to a transformation of consciousness.

In the chapters ahead, we shall witness firsthand this awakening as it has occurred in several of my patients, and perhaps even marvel when we perceive how a deeper intelligence, ostensibly dormant until their awakening, seemed to have been guiding their lives all along.

My hope is that these stories and the accumulated wisdom I share in these pages will serve you well, most especially if you yourself, or a loved one of yours, have been dually-diagnosed. This book is also written to help health professionals – be they physicians, psychologists, nurses, counselors, social workers or other "healers" – to better understand dual diagnosis and the treatment alternatives.

CHAPTER 1

DUAL DIAGNOSIS UNVEILED

"The mind is everything:
what you think, you become."

– Gautama Buddha

"To one who has faith, no explanation is necessary.
To one without faith, no explanation is possible."

– St. Thomas Aquinas

This book is about dual diagnosis, a medical condition that occurs by definition when both a chemical dependency and some form of mental illness affect the same individual at the same time. Each side of the equation includes symptoms that interfere with the person's ability to function effectively. However, not only is that individual affected by two separate illnesses, but these interact synergistically: by this I mean that each disorder exacerbates the other and also predisposes to relapse in the other. At times, the symptoms can overlap or even mask each other, making diagnosis and treatment all the more difficult.

Dual diagnosis is becoming increasingly prevalent in Canada. There are estimates that up to .28% of the Canadian population may be afflicted – over 90,000 Canadians. [1] And yet, rather surprisingly, the topic has received little if any attention from the popular press. There is a vast quantity of media coverage on addiction and on mental illness separately, but only rare articles or features concerning both subjects as they occur concurrently within the same individual.

How mental illness presents within the milieu of addiction is a complex phenomenon. The association reflects the interchange of a myriad of influences that I will shortly outline. As well, the admixture of an individual's ideas, attitudes, beliefs and values – colloquially referred to as his or her "belief system" – plays a definite and central role. To be more exact, how well an individual is coping with his or her illness at any particular moment is directly impacted by the inherent stability of his or her belief system.

I have already mentioned that dual diagnosis affects an estimated .28% of the Canadian population. While this figure may already seem high, what is more surprising yet is that due to greater awareness and vigilance, the condition is being diagnosed and treated at greater frequency in adolescents. This in turn suggests that early childhood experiences play a critical role in the presentation and development of illness.

Despite recent studies [2] indicating that adolescent drug use, and alcohol use in particular, have remained essentially stable, adolescent substance abuse remains a concern overall because it can contribute to the development of subsequent mental health issues. This evidence also suggests that some people use alcohol or other drugs of abuse in part to self-medicate distressing mental states associated with underlying psychiatric conditions.

Whether the chicken came first or the egg, adolescents with substance use disorders (SUDs), like adults, exhibit a higher rate of psychiatric problems as compared to the general population. Some of the following conditions, including Attention Deficit Disorder (ADD), are seen preferentially in adolescents, whereas others, like schizophrenia, are found more in the adult population. The following is a list of mental illnesses commonly associated with SUD:

- Anxiety disorders
- Depressive disorders
- Attention Deficit Disorder (ADD)
- Bipolar Disorder
- Conduct Disorder and other Cluster B personality disorders
- Obsessive Compulsive Disorder (OCD)
- Schizophrenia

Certain factors put children and adolescents at risk for developing a substance usage disorder. These include:

Genetic factors

- Having one or both parents with a substance abuse problem

Constitutional and psychological factors

- Psychiatric problems
- History of physical, sexual or emotional abuse
- History of attempted suicide

Sociological and cultural factors

- Family
- Parental experiences with and attitudes towards drug use
- History of parental divorce or separation
- Low expectations for the child

Peers

- Friends who use drugs
- Friends' attitudes towards drug use
- Antisocial or delinquent behavior

School

- Failing or dropping out

Community

- Community attitudes towards drug use
- Economic and social deprivation
- Availability of alcohol and drugs (including tobacco in cigarettes)

As a counterbalance to these many factors, and despite them, having an entrenched belief system helps to create stability in a person's life. [3] It enables the individual to process his or her life experiences at a deeper level of awareness, to own these experiences, and to sometimes even experience a natural state of euphoria colloquially called "bliss." Without a strong belief system, the same person could just as easily fall prey to the many ill effects of instability including dysfunctional relationships of all kinds, financial failure, jail, institutionalization and premature death.

For the average individual suffering the ill effects of a substance use disorder, whether in conjunction with a mental illness or not, the typical recuperative route to follow is to join a self-help group or fellowship such as Alcoholics Anonymous or its equivalent. Such programs strengthen the fledgling belief system of the individual and provide structure. Working within the framework, the person becomes capable in time of assuming responsibility for his or her own spiritual growth. Support groups of this kind also expressly encourage the development of altruism within the individual by assisting addicts to work with one another and begin navigating the complexities of healthy relationships under the tutelage of more senior members of the group.

There is a strong component of "sin and salvation" involved in many of these programs, which suggests many would be replacing one form of dependency (drugs, alcohol, etc.) with another, albeit more benign, one. Yet I would argue that augmenting an ounce of brimstone and damnation fear with a pound of dogmatic faith may not be the best long-term therapy. A far more useful proposition would be to eliminate the fear. I believe that the only way to do this is through self-knowledge. Ultimately, whether one chooses to believe in a personal God should be a matter of choice and preference, not dread.

As an aside, the "sin and salvation" approach emphasizes that Adam and Eve disobeyed God when they ate of the fruit of the Tree of Knowledge in the Garden of Eden and were banished from Paradise. Yet that Knowledge has ultimately facilitated the triumphant return of humankind to the open arms of God. The parable of the Fall is thus a powerful symbol for the return to wholeness. A more contemporary rendition is coming to terms with what Carl Jung called the "Shadow." [4]

In my opinion, Jung's concept of Shadow throws light on the spiritual dimension of dual diagnosis. Why? Because at some point, individuals with a dual diagnosis must ask themselves, "Who am I?" This generally occurs sometime after the stirring of consciousness within, and it marks the transition from mundane thought to a state of awareness. Paradoxically, it is at this particular juncture that formal belief systems break down for many people, and the individual will typically seek out the services of a priest or counselor, a modern-day shaman or some other spiritual healer or guide.

To be more explicit, Jung's concept of the Shadow comes into play when an individual has not yet reconciled his or her natural polarities and experiences inner turmoil or conflict because of the divergent forces battling for supremacy within. This can lead, in and of itself, to a whole range of disorders that give rise to a dual diagnosis.

Some risk factors concerning dual diagnosis have been listed, but what specific behavioral clues should one be on the lookout for? *The Diagnostic and Statistical Manual of Mental Disorders - IV* defines "substance abusers" as people who persist in using mood-altering substances despite recurrent social, interpersonal and legal problems as a result of their drug use. "Harmful use" or "dependency" (further along the spectrum of substance abuse) implies drug use that causes either physical or mental damage. People who have become chemically dependent meet all of the criteria for being substance abusers, but will also exhibit some or all of the following traits:

- Narrowing of the substance repertoire (using only one brand or type of substance)
- Drink- or drug-seeking behavior (only going to social events that will include use of the chosen substance, or only hanging out with others who use)
- Tolerance (having to use increasing amounts to achieve the same effect)
- Withdrawal symptoms (experiencing symptoms of physical discomfort after going a short period without using)
- Using to relieve or avoid withdrawal symptoms (such as using to stop the shakes or "cure" a hangover)
- A subjective awareness of the compulsion to use or the craving for a substance (whether admitted to someone else or not)
- A return to using after a period of abstinence (deciding to quit and not being able to follow through)

Checking "yes" to three or more of the foregoing criteria is strongly suggestive of the presence of a Substance Use Disorder (SUD). Typically, those who are diagnosed as "substance abusers only" (still rather early on along the spectrum of substance abuse) can be helped with a brief intervention, including education concerning the dangers of binge use and substance poisoning. Those who have become "substance-dependent" generally require outside help to stop using, which could include detoxification, medical treatment, institutionalization, counseling and/or self-help group support such as Alcoholics Anonymous. Note that once an individual becomes substance dependent, they cannot then regress and become substance abusers at a later time by definition. This is simply because abstinence remains the goal of medical management; at least over the intermediate term.

What about the mental illness component of a dual diagnosis? Although there is a wide range of possible disorders, some typical "flavors" are presented here. Available evidence [5] suggests that certain mental illnesses tend to be characteristically associated with chemical dependency. Those listed earlier in this chapter will be briefly discussed below.

Anxiety disorders, for example, are among the most common psychiatric conditions co-existing in both adolescents and adults with a substance use disorder. Typical manifestations include **Post Traumatic Stress Disorder** (PTSD), **Social Phobia** and **Generalized Anxiety Disorder**.

Before we continue, a slight digression is in order here concerning adolescents. Many teenagers believe, as many adults do, that drugs and alcohol can reduce anxiety and stress, and this may lead to first use or continued abuse. This does not mean that drug use actually does prevent anxiety. In fact, there are well-founded studies [6] showing that teenagers who never experiment with drugs or alcohol may be at higher risk of developing anxiety problems later in life.

It stands to reason that a young person with a mental health problem such as an anxiety disorder may elect not to engage in social experiments involving drugs, and may tend to stay away from peers who do. However, should an anxiety disorder develop to the point of becoming entrenched, this does not prevent the subject from developing an SUD later. What causes what is the subject of our next chapter.

To carry on with our list of mental disorders that can co-exist with a Substance Use Disorder, both adolescents and adults are at great risk for developing a **Depressive Disorder** or *dysthymia* ("minor" depression). Clinical practitioners are often faced with a chicken-or-egg dilemma in attempting to determine which came first; the mental illness and then the SUD, or vice versa.

Of note, for adults, depressive symptoms oftentimes resolve within a few weeks of the person "drying out" or abstaining from drugs or alcohol. Yet in adolescents this is rarely the case. Depressive symptoms in younger people often require treatment with antidepressants. Moreover, one of the greatest risk factors for teen suicide is intoxication with either drugs or alcohol.[7]

Current research evidence [8] shows that treatment with serotonin-augmenting medications or "atypical" antidepressants has proven effective. When drugs within different classes are combined to improve the overall antidepressant activity, it is rarely necessary to augment the dosages. Additionally, individual psychotherapy may be part of the treatment plan recommended by the psychiatrist or mental health team.

Attention Deficit Disorder (ADD) is the most common psychiatric disorder diagnosed. It affects from 3% to 5% of people globally. The term ADD can be used interchangeably with the older term ADHD (Attention Deficit Hyperactivity Disorder). Scientific findings [9] confirm that pre- and post-natal stresses are the most important determinants of this condition in children. The impact of early stress on the brain – when the mother is depressed, for example – creates vulnerability to ADD and to addictions.

Children with ADD who are not on medication typically have an attention span of a few seconds only. They are disruptive in class and generally exhibit behavioral problems both in the home and at school. It is perhaps no wonder that as they grow up, they tend to gravitate towards experimentation with substances of potential abuse.

The treatments of choice are psychostimulants such as Ritalin or Dexedrine, which can be a concern as both drugs are amphetamines (commonly known as "speed") and have the potential to be abused. Luckily, alternate medications do exist. Furthermore, it has recently been suggested [10] that appropriate treatment of ADD may lead to a decreased chance of developing a substance usage disorder.

In his highly-recommended book *Scattered Minds*, [10] Dr. Gabor Maté talks candidly about the condition of ADD. Dr. Maté has himself been diagnosed with ADD and is living proof that there is help – and the prospect of a healthy, productive life – for individuals suffering from this often-debilitating condition.

Bipolar Disorder is a tricky diagnosis to make in the presence of co-existing addiction, but in substance-abusing teens, it is complicated even further. Behaviors such as changes in sleeping patterns and mood swings can be symptomatic of this illness, substance abuse, or even normal adolescence. Diagnosis of Bipolar Disorder should certainly be a consideration as concerns substance-abusing youth, particularly those with a binge pattern. Treatment is often complex, and can be extended to include medications and psychotherapy once stability is achieved.

Conduct Disorder (formerly known as **Antisocial Personality Disorder** or APD) is another manifestation classified medically as a personality disorder. Prevalence varies from 1% to 4% in children between the ages of 9 and 17 depending upon how the disorder is defined. It can affect substance abusing teenagers, and is more frequently diagnosed in boys than girls. [11] The disorder is also more common in urban than in rural populations. [12]

The pathognomonic feature of Conduct Disorder is aggressive behavior associated with a flagrant disregard for the law and the rights of others. Conduct Disorder that persists beyond the age of 18 is frequently diagnosed as Antisocial Personality Disorder. Whatever the age of onset, Conduct Disorder is often difficult if not impossible to treat effectively.

Perhaps the highest risk for the association of a problem with either drugs or alcohol and a mental health problem occurs in individuals with *both* Conduct Disorder and a mood disorder (either Unipolar Depression or Bipolar Disorder). Impulse control is an aspect of self-regulation, and affected individuals generally have problems with both. Disordered self-regulation, in this case, is a phenomenon whereby the cerebral cortex, which typically permits or overrides impulses from traveling from the lower brain centers, does not function optimally. As in Bipolar Disorder, diagnosis and treatment are often complex issues. For this reason, youth with a combination of Conduct Disorder and an SUD frequently require long-term residential treatment.

The other so-called **Cluster B personality disorders** (typically associated together as a group because they exhibit a predilection towards dramatic or erratic behaviors) tend to be characteristically associated with a Substance

Use Disorder. This group includes: **Narcissistic Personality Disorder, Borderline Personality Disorder** and **Histrionic Personality Disorder**, all of which tend to be diagnosed later in life. We shall examine these disorders at greater length in future chapters.

Obsessive Compulsive Disorder (OCD) is the fourth most commonly diagnosed mental disorder, affecting from 1% to 2% of the Canadian population. It is an anxiety disorder that has important features in common with addiction, so the underlying mechanisms that govern OCD deserve some explanation.

We tend to believe that we are in control of the decisions we make, but they can also stem at times from emotional drives or subliminal beliefs of which we are not consciously aware. The stronger a person's automatic brain mechanisms and the weaker the part of the brain that imposes conscious control, the less true freedom the individual will be able to exercise in his or her life choices.

When overcome by stress or overwhelming emotions, almost any human will act or react not from intent or free will but from a quasi-instinctual or less-than-fully autonomous impulses stemming from more primitive or instinctual drives deep within the brain. Though these mechanisms are not entirely understood at this time, it is believed that in the case of OCD, the cerebral cortex, the part of the brain that houses volitional functions, does not self-regulate to the degree apparent in other vital processes like the regulation of blood pressure and the control of heart rate, for example. The referral mechanisms that oversee and govern self-regulation are somehow short-circuited and the necessary feedback is no longer available for the afflicted subject to act with conscious intent.

People with OCD experience both obsessions and compulsions. Obsessions are unwanted and disturbing thoughts, images or impulses that suddenly pop into the mind and cause a great deal of anxiety or distress. Compulsions are deliberate behaviors (such as repeated hand-washing, checking on miscellaneous things or putting them in order) or mental acts (praying or chanting, counting, repeating word phrases and such) that are carried out repeatedly to reduce the anxiety caused by the obsessions. Over time, OCD symptoms can change. For example, a subject may start off washing his or her hands compulsively, but later develop excessive checking behaviors and stop compulsive hand-washing altogether.

Young adults between the ages of 18 and 24 are at highest risk for developing OCD. However, many adults with the disease say their symptoms started when they were children or adolescents. Men tend to develop OCD at an earlier age (usually between the ages of 14 and 19.5 years) than do women (usually between the ages of 21 and 22). Among adults, women report having OCD slightly more frequently than men. [13]

Left untreated, OCD is a debilitating illness. The disease is best treated medically with a class of antidepressants called serum serotonin reuptake inhibitors (SSRI's). Many people with anxiety disorders such as OCD benefit from joining a self-help or support group and sharing their problems and achievements with others.

Stress management techniques and meditation can help people with anxiety disorders to calm themselves and may enhance the effects of therapy. There is preliminary evidence [14] that aerobic exercise can also have a calming effect. Since caffeine, certain illicit drugs and even some over-the-counter cold medications can aggravate the symptoms of anxiety disorders, they should be avoided.

Schizophrenia is another prevalent disorder, affecting about 1% of Canadians or 1 in 100 people. Currently, about 52% of admissions for schizophrenia to general hospitals are for adults from the ages of 25 to 44, and the rates are increasing among young and middle-aged men. The disease also tends to be more severe in men than in women.

Most cases of schizophrenia appear in the late teens or early adulthood. For men, the average age of onset is 25. For women, it is around the age of 30. However schizophrenia can also appear for the first time in middle age or even later. In rare cases, it can even affect young children and adolescents, although the symptoms manifest slightly differently than they do in adults. In general, the earlier schizophrenia develops, the more severe it is.

The 2002 Academy Award winner for Best Picture, *A Beautiful Mind*, brought schizophrenia into the public eye by portraying how the illness progressed in the life of John Forbes Nash, Jr., the 1994 Nobel Prize laureate in Economics. [15] As the film illustrates, schizophrenia makes it difficult for a person to distinguish between what is real and what is unreal, to think clearly and to behave in socially acceptable ways. These obstacles can have a severe impact on one's work, relationships and day-to-day functioning. But with treatment and support, as the film also depicted, a person with schizophrenia can still lead a productive life.

Families with mentally ill relatives whose problems are compounded by substance abuse face problems of enormous proportions. Mental health services are not well prepared to deal with patients having both afflictions. Often only one of the two problems is identified. If both are recognized, the individual may be bounced back and forth between services for mental illness and those for addiction, or worse, the person may be refused treatment by both agencies. The picture to date has not been rosy, but there are signs that dual diagnosis is now being recognized as such, and an increasing number of programs are trying to address the treatment needs of people with a combination of problems.

Research studies [16] are beginning to help us understand the scope of the problem. It is now generally agreed that as much as 50% of the mentally ill population also has a substance abuse problem. The drug most commonly used is alcohol, followed by marijuana and cocaine. Prescription drugs such as tranquilizers and sleeping medications are also likely candidates. The incidence of abuse is greatest among males and those from ages 18 to 44. Substance abuse complicates almost every aspect of care for a person with mental illness.

In its very comprehensive 2008 Position Paper [17], the National Coalition on Dual Diagnosis reported that people with a dual diagnosis:

- Have complex needs and find themselves entangled in multiple in-depth systems of assessment and management, often unconnected to one another
- Have inadequate access to positive determinants of health (education, housing, nutrition, economic security, work, safe communities and social inclusion)
- Experience the double jeopardy that arises when two disabilities (developmental and/or mental health needs) occur within the same individual, making diagnostic overshadowing more likely. (This means that some symptoms are trivialized or relegated to the status of a developmental problem rather than being recognized as a legitimate mental health concern. As a result, the afflicted person becomes even more marginalized.) Substance abuse within this context simply increases the complexity of the issues involved
- Are more likely than their non-disabled peers to exhibit challenging behaviors such as self-mutilation, aggression, non-compliance or other

destructive and disruptive behaviors that increase social stigma and further compound the marginalization

- Tend to be over-medicated with psychotropic medications to quell their "acting out" behaviors without an in-depth assessment of the underlying reasons why they occur.

What can and should society do? Homelessness, the provision of comprehensive medical services and the containment of infectious diseases, such as tuberculosis, hepatitis and AIDS, are some of the more visible complex social problems today associated with Canada's dually diagnosed population and sub-populations (those who have developmental rather than mental health issues per se). As has been mentioned, however, possibly .28% of adult Canadians struggle with a dual diagnosis (as defined at the outset of the chapter), which represents a significant challenge for society in general and for those afflicted. These individuals could benefit from greater community resources in general and from Harm Reduction incentives in particular that will be covered in later chapters.

Many of the problems we have been discussing are stereotyped as afflicting mainly a down-and-out fringe element of society. Relief organizations such as the Roman Catholic Church and the Salvation Army seem to do some good amongst this element because, despite the evangelical streak that may accompany their services, they do attempt to minister to such individuals based on compassion rather than antagonism. But for society as a whole to truly address the root causes of poverty, hunger, mental illness and addiction in a meaningful and effective way, I believe that the upper strata of our society needs to be mobilized to look the issues straight in the eye and realize that many of the downtrodden do not choose their fate. Were decison-makers' eyes truly open, they would realize, no matter what their outward convictions, that "There, but for the grace of God, go I."

One can imagine how quickly things could change for the better if a majority of Canadians acknowledged and mobilized to send an unambiguous message to the federal government in Ottawa that the right-wing political agenda being advanced today is serving only the privileged few while the many face narrowing horizons, and a growing number of Canadians are falling, disenfranchised, through the cracks.

Unfettered free-market economics have served only to spend our children's birthright, polarize society and entrench a self-righteous entitlement mentality in the halls of power. Materialism is eroding the common decency at the heart of Canadian society and undermining our deep-set compassion for the underdog.

One traditional index of a society's wealth is the standard of health care afforded its citizens. Canada is a wealthy nation today because social democracy has been the reigning political platform for most of our recent political history. Come election time, let us not forget that the health of our people is Canada's most precious resource, and that our social programs, so dearly won, are a beacon of sanity in a dark world today. Let us not be fooled or intimidated into relinquishing them under the flimsy guise of economic reform. Safeguarding our health is not a question of money, and failure is not an option. Otherwise, the short end of the stick will prove to be very long indeed.

CHAPTER 2

THE MASKS OF DUAL DIAGNOSIS

"Oh, life is a glorious cycle of song,
A medley of extemporanea;
And love is a thing that can never go wrong;
And I am Marie of Romania."

– Dorothy Parker

Having introduced two central topics in the last chapter – dual diagnosis and the importance of belief systems in dealing with it – I now wish to discuss the symptoms of dually diagnosed patients, paying particular attention to how an individual's stability is impacted by the quality of his or her beliefs.

But first, let me discuss possible origins of the condition. Rather than simple cause and effect, the relationship between mental illness and substance abuse is in fact extremely complex. Consider four possible scenarios:

1. Mental illness "causes" substance use. (The individual self-medicates to quell the symptoms of the disorder.)

2. Substance use "causes" mental illness. (Substance abuse triggers

neurochemical alterations, stress and demoralization that eventually lead to full-blown mental disorder.)

3. There is common causality. (Something else causes both conditions such as genetics, the environment, etc.)

4. There is no causal relationship. (It is common for the conditions to co-exist and neither causes the other.)

Before we can determine which are more likely scenarios, it is appropriate to begin with a discussion of the underlying dynamics of mental illness during infancy and early childhood development. Why? Because this will lead us to discuss the topic of boundaries, and, as we shall see, boundaries tie in directly with the notion of belief systems, which in turn begin to form quite early in life.

Before birth, there is a conspicuous absence of a physical boundary between the fetus and its mother. This changes abruptly and irrevocably with birth. Research into intra-uterine experiences suggests that trauma sustained at this crucial moment may have lasting ramifications, but the degree to which birth memories are retained is still subject to controversy.

It is generally accepted that in early infancy, the child remains enmeshed with its parental figures, meaning that it does not yet perceive any boundaries. At each successive stage of the developmental process, the immature ego progressively differentiates itself from its attachment figures, the child begins to explore how it is indeed separate from its parents, and the idea of "self" is consolidated. During this period, the infant also acquires a rudimentary sense of "good" and "bad." As early developmental experiences and events unfold, the child ideally learns to construct a healthy self-image with appropriate feedback from the parental figures.

An integral function of a healthy immature ego is the identification of both healthy boundaries and limits. A sense of self and a sense of one's boundaries seem to go hand in hand. The mature counterpart to the immature or libidinal ego encompasses one's capacity for critical thought as well as one's aggressive tendencies and basic sense of sexuality – in short, one's survival instincts. The mature ego, ideally, as normal development proceeds is relegated to serve as a point of reference. It functions basically like radar, screening external events and processing them internally.

In families where boundary distortions are the rule, parents continue to project negatively upon each other and upon the child. In turn, the child continues to perceive him- or herself as an extension of the parents, and the enmeshment issue remains unresolved. As the child gets older, inappropriate mirroring or "feedback" by the parents can furnish inappropriate cues as to what is "good" and "bad," thereby setting the stage for developmental problems down the road.

If the parental figures continue to role model inappropriately, the child will already perceive him- or herself as "different" from other children such that by about the age of two pathology is evident to the trained eye, and henceforth the child will begin to exhibit prominent dysfunctional traits. Children raised in a dysfunctional setting typically have difficulty setting boundaries, experiencing appropriate levels of self-esteem and knowing who they are. Not surprisingly, they are prone to role-playing, as they tend to carry a lot of the family's emotional weight.

Whatever the age at which the complications of mental illness begin to appear, they exhibit across a continuum, at the far end of which is psychosis requiring drug treatment and long-term institutionalization. What exactly is psychosis? The simplest definition is *losing touch with reality*. Substance abuse is one of the commonest causes of psychosis. Others include illness, infection and brain injury. It is important to identify psychosis early because it is treatable. When it is left untreated, neurotoxicity occurs [i.e. natural and/or artificial substances which are toxic to the nervous system cause damage to the nervous tissue, including the brain] and treatment outcomes are poor due to resistance to the usual agents or irreversible neuron damage.

In the last half-century, there has been a shift in medical thinking from a psychodynamic to a neurobiological understanding of mental illness. In other words, it is not "all in the mind." Matter counts too. The discovery of the opiate receptor centers of the brain in the 1950s was just one in a string of conceptual advances that helped to consolidate this shift. Another contributing factor was the serendipitous discovery of the first anti-psychotic medication, chlorpromazine, which was originally introduced as a surgical anesthetic.

The fate of behaviorally-disturbed psychotic patients prior to the discovery of these so-called neuroleptic agents was involuntary committal and institutionalization. Although a very select few individuals responded somewhat to psychotherapy, it was not a practical solution to the problem of agitation within the acutely behaviorally disturbed psychotic patient.

Second-generation neuroleptic agents like clozapine have fewer harmful side-effects. They act on dopamine receptors in the brain, which, together with other neurotransmitters, govern the manifestation of psychoses, including both hallucinations and delusions.

A hallucination is a misperception. These may be auditory or visual, though the auditory form is by far the more common. A delusion is a false belief. Again, there are various themes, which are characteristically related to a particular mental illness. For example, religious delusions are often seen in manic-depressive people with psychosis whereas persecutory or bizarre delusions are often seen in people with schizophrenia.

A newer generation of "atypical" anti-psychotic agents was introduced in the 1970s to treat psychosis, and since that time, newer and safer agents have come on the market. The main side effects of these so-called "second generation agents" are weight gain leading to metabolic complications, which in turn can lead to diabetes and possible cardiovascular complications.

The paradigm shift that occurred about a half-century ago has revolutionized the understanding and management of neurobiological mental illnesses. I am not sure however that this development is entirely for the better because the newer neuroleptic agents do not address the underlying psychodynamics of mental illness alluded to earlier when I discussed early childhood development. They deal instead with a superficial understanding of these conditions. To my mind, this is one reason why clinical stability takes so long to achieve, and I will support my argument with clinical cases shortly.

Having introduced the topic of causation and contributory factors to dual diagnosis at the outset of the chapter, let me now discuss in more detail each of the four basic scenarios presented earlier. The first suggests that mental illness causes substance abuse, presumably through some mechanism involving self-medication. In the following case study, it plays a key role.

"Rob" has a long history of depression dating back to his teens. He did not self-medicate these early episodes, but in his early 20's, he sought medical help and was started on antidepressant therapy. Within months, the medication unmasked his underlying mania and he became floridly psychotic. In laymen's terms, he "lost it." For example, he began spending uncontrollably, turned promiscuous, and was ultimately incarcerated for drunk driving. He was then hospitalized, but as he was crafty enough to evade the appropriate diagnosis, he returned to regular life and his mania continued.

After three years, he was again hospitalized when his colleagues at work complained of strange behaviors on his part. This time, a diagnosis of Bipolar Type 1 Depression (with psychosis) was conferred. "Rob" was started on medication and did well for some time. However, he did not follow up properly with medical care and did not take his medication regularly, and began abusing alcohol in order to self-medicate his symptoms. When he was hospitalized for the third time, a further two years hence, both elements of his diagnosis were addressed. It took five years from initial hospitalization to the final conferment of his dual diagnosis. Today "Rob" is five years clean and sober and he remains for the most part stable on medication.

Why is "Rob" stable? Is it simply because he takes his medication regularly? He himself says, "Call it what you will. I call it faith. I believe 'God' is directing my life and I simply have a hand to play in it." This supports my contention as a long-time clinical observer that an individual's belief system greatly affects his or her stabilization.

Let us now look at the second scenario, where substance abuse is said to cause mental illness, presumably by inducing stress, demoralization and neurochemical alterations. In the next case history, the role of medication is again clear cut, but its effect is somewhat tenuous.

"Kristopher" has Schizoaffective Disorder, a hybrid condition combining some of the elements of schizophrenia and a mood disorder that is not often encountered in general practice. As it turns out, "Kristopher" began abusing substances in his early teens, using mainly pot and LSD socially with friends. At a later stage, he would use anything he could get his hands on, which included crack cocaine, crystal methamphetamine and Ecstasy. He was diagnosed with Schizoaffective Disorder at the age of 24, after being mislabeled by two different psychiatrists initially and placed on medication. Despite treatment, his social functioning remains marginal. Furthermore, though he now sees the drugs he used in the past as "bad," he still continues to drink and he smokes pot regularly.

It would seem that scenario 2, in which substance abuse causes mental illness, does have some bearing on "Kristopher's" case. He has lost the ability to think for himself, needs constant direction, and more or less functions like a machine. The medical term for this is "pickling." The relevant question is why "Kristopher" ended up this way instead of stabilizing into a more productive life. Let's look at his belief system.

"Kristopher's" mother got pregnant in her early teens. He knows little if anything about his biological father. Raised as a Methodist by his grandparents, he now dabbles in the occult in his spare time. As his treating physician, I posit that in order to keep out of harm's way, ingesting fairly lofty doses of antipsychotic medication is his best defense.

Is there hope for "Kristopher"? These days, he is toying with the idea of giving up alcohol and pot altogether. I have told him that I fully support him in this decision. His main problem is that he is a bit of a recluse. Were he to stop isolating himself and establish a circle of support, he would be greatly aided in his endeavor. He is genuinely likeable, but he lacks self-confidence and he harbors a lot of resentment toward his orthodox religious upbringing. This, however, is not altogether a bad sign: at least he believes, if not acknowledges, there is a God.

The role of psychosocial therapy in "Kristopher's" case would be to help him consolidate his beliefs in order that they work for him, rather than against him. I firmly believe having seen countless cases like this one that once this consolidation is accomplished and he begins to own his experiences, he can be guided along an appropriate path and ultimately achieve stability in his life. One proof of stabilization would be a growing ability on his part to successfully navigate the difficult area of personal relationships.

At this point, we might ask whether addiction itself is a disease. There is a growing body of evidence in support of this fact. [1] I myself believe that where addiction precedes the onset of mental illness, environmental issues need to be addressed and measures need to be taken to confront the problem of addiction. These may include detoxification, residential treatment and/or psychotherapy.

Let us now look at the third scenario, one which posits that one or more common causes underlie both the mental illness component and the substance abuse leading to abuse including such things as genetic and environmental factors.

"Michael" has been a patient of mine for some time. When he first came to see me, he was not living on the street, but he had gotten involved with the drug subculture and contracted a heroin habit that was costing $80 to $100 a day. He was soliciting as a male prostitute in order to satisfy his dependency.

After a few sessions, "Michael" said something that struck me as quite odd: "A bird in the bush is worth two in hand!" In time, as we developed a therapeutic relationship and he came to appreciate the notion of healthy boundaries, I asked him how many sexual partners he had had. When he told me he was a closet bisexual, I finally understood his strange remark. I also realized that he had not yet come to terms with his sexuality. Today, "Michael" leads an openly gay lifestyle. Let's look at his history in a little more detail. He comments:

I grew up in an extremely religious household. During my childhood, I recall my parents being rather harsh disciplinarians. Despite the fact that their marriage was stable, it was extremely turbulent. My father was an alcoholic – though he was in recovery when he met my mom – and there is a strong family history of mental illness on her side. She was emotionally abusive, particularly towards my father. Not only that, but my mother has a history of severe depression. In fact, she was depressed during her pregnancy with me.

Early in recovery, "Michael" was diagnosed with hepatitis C, which he acquired through injection drug use. Around this time, he was also diagnosed with Attention Deficit Disorder (ADD). Both issues have somewhat complicated his recovery. He is now on a methadone program and follows up regularly with me. He has supervised urine drug screening which has been negative apart from methadone metabolites for many months, and has now attained sufficient stability that he can be treated for his hepatitis C. He has also graduated from regularly supervised to random monitoring of his urine.

Methadone is a synthetic opiate antagonist that is used therapeutically to combat heroin addiction. Due to the long half-life of the drug (meaning that it persists in the blood stream for quite a while), it can be dosed once a day. This makes it possible for addicts to lead productive, stable lives without having to shoot up several times a day, and without diverting their time and energy into searching for ways to procure their next fix. Typically, an individual is started on a low dose of the drug, and it is incrementally raised until all cravings for opiates have subsided. Participants may choose to stay on the program or wean themselves off methadone as they see fit under medical supervision.

Today, "Michael" holds down a steady job and is going to school part-time to earn a diploma in electronic business systems management. He is also in a stable monogamous relationship. He got married earlier this year to "Greg." Apart from being significantly older and more tolerant, "Greg" is also patient and understanding. The two make a handsome couple.

All this would not have been possible were it not for the methadone and the psychostimulant medication "Michael" takes for his ADD. Moreover, he has come out of the closet and has developed a value system of his own that he abides by. Curiously enough, he has adopted some of the values of his childhood such as marriage and a belief in a Higher Power. He has managed to counterbalance both genetic and environmental factors in his recovery thanks in part I would contend to the stability within the home and the values he imbibed during childhood.

Now for the final scenario, the one where the two conditions of mental illness and substance abuse are associated in the absence of a common cause. Let's look at how this can occur.

"Jaspreet" recently started using cocaine. As is common, this habit started through peer pressure. Her boyfriend dealt the drug, which made it easily accessible to her. However, the relationship was abusive, and she came in to see me because she was experiencing symptoms of depression. During our first visit, she informed me she was scared of her boyfriend and did not know how to get out of the relationship. On numerous occasions, he had threatened to harm her if she left.

I started "Jaspreet" on anti-depressant medication, which worked marvelously, and also recommended that she look into drug rehab and find a safe house for battered women. She followed up on this advice. Within six months, she was no longer clinically depressed, was off the cocaine, and had made strides towards a new beginning. Her antidepressant was tapered over the next several months.

The about-face in "Jaspreet's" circumstances leads me to introduce another point about the remarks I make. I work in two addiction clinics, one in downtown Vancouver and the other in a large suburb of the city. In the downtown clinic, I see a lot of co-existing physical disorders, particularly sexually transmitted diseases (STDs), HIV-related illnesses and hepatitis. There is also a higher rate of serious mental illnesses in the downtown population.

In the suburban clinic, I deal mainly with migrant workers who work extremely long hours doing menial jobs. Their addiction is a function of the type of work they do, the long hours they work and the existing social fabric. Many of my patients from this group have a stable family life and belong to the Sikh religious community, which has an extensive social network. I contend that the basic infrastructure that is in place within this community reduces the existence of so-called comorbid conditions (such as HIV-related illnesses, severe mental illnesses and such) and speaks to the need for an entrenched system of values which individuals may imbibe as this confers a predilection toward stability over the intermediate and long term.

Cross-cultural comparison between the two populations reveals that within the sub-population of individuals in the downtown core, in addition to the usual environmental factors, genetic factors are no doubt operative in the majority of cases. This leads me to conclude that so-called genetic factors may only come into play once the usual safeguards such as psychosocial stability conferred within the home and the immediate microenvironment have begun to erode and no longer provide an adaptive advantage. The issue we are dealing with within the subpopulation of individuals within the downtown core is primarily trauma, particularly neo-natal and early developmental trauma. In contrast, within the suburban community and despite some exceptions, the crux of the problem seems to be an inability to erect and maintain meaningful boundaries, which are oftentimes inbred manifesting if you will as innate cultural phenomena. My point here is to suggest that psychodynamics when viewed socially if not individually do play an important role despite the paradigm shift which has occurred over the last half century or so in favor of a strictly neurobiologic explanation of both certain mental illnesses and related addictive behaviors. Therefore, it is important to weigh psychosocial factors and their potential contribution to the overall management plan in individuals conferred with a dual diagnosis.

It is well known [2] that childhood abuse, and in particular a history of sexual abuse, can lead to the onset of both mental illness and addictive illness later in life. Cultural factors can be equally important in some contexts even though they may surface less often or appear less severe. For example, in some societies, individual expression is virtually submerged by the larger cultural identity when the community, clan or tribe comes first. It is important to consider and weigh the possible effects of cultural factors in dual diagnosis particularly as concerns the more common anxiety and mood disorders which often coexist within the milieu of a Substance Use Disorder. I say this simply because it has been my experience that particularly in the case of anxiety disorders, they tend to predate the onset of an associated SUD. The key point here is prevention of a SUD.

To end our discussion of possible causes, let us now turn to what recourse is available, and in particular, to Harm Reduction as a philosophy of reform. Harm Reduction is based on the recognition that people always have engaged, and always will engage, in risky behaviors including casual sex, prostitution and/or drug use. The main objective of Harm Reduction is to mitigate the potential dangers and health risks associated with the risky behaviors themselves rather than attempting to eradicate the behaviors themselves. As a public-health strategy, it is intended to be a progressive alternative to the outright prohibition of potentially dangerous lifestyle choices.

And what belief system have I personally evolved? When it comes to spirituality, I seek authenticity over and above all else in my life. I do not necessarily believe something because I have read it or because some authority states that it is so. What I consider to be infallible is that which I myself have lived and know to be true. The truth speaks for itself. If I were to sum up "my" religion in one word, that word would be "faith."

When I am asked what faith is, however, my response is always, "Why are you asking me? Ask yourself!" I do not believe there is any single "correct" answer. Faith is something, like intuition, that everyone possesses and that is important to cultivate. Why? Faith will not help a person change water into wine or walk across water, but it can move mountains when that person comes to believe that God is doing what he or she cannot. An inner transformation occurs. Call it an awakening.

The traditional medical paradigm treats only the periphery of dual diagnosis. In order to achieve stability, I believe that spiritual clarity must be part of the treatment. Faith and self-knowledge are two possible paths to get to it, and at the end of the road, the light of consciousness beckons along with the beacon of love.

I believe there is such a thing as spiritual love or *agape*. It is love devoid of any carnal aspect, which is a concept the dually-diagnosed sometimes have trouble comprehending as they are frequently plagued with sex problems. Most individuals with a dual diagnosis confuse love with attachment. The even deeper issue is the psychological dependency at the root of the attachment. Under-lying all is the ego and its paralyzing, toxic fear. If love was understood and embraced within our Western society as being primarily spiritual rather than carnal I would contend that a lot of the difficulties in comprehending the term would be obviated. However, as it stands this is perhaps wishful thinking be-cause today "love" whether defined in positive or negative terms has become something which is little more than a commodity and as such remains a fantasy at least for the vast majority of our younger generation particularly the dually diagnosed.

At the end of the day, it all boils down to a question of boundaries. When sound boundaries are in place, we may then know, protect and experience our true selves. We can vanquish the fear. But for that to happen, we need to relin-quish control, the basic mandate of the ego, and surrender to the reality. With less compulsion and anxiety about running the show, things go the way they are meant to in life, which is often better than good, thanks to the grace of a God of one's own understanding.

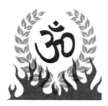

THE SCOPE OF THE PROBLEM

"The more choices you have, the more your values matter."

– Michael Schrage

"If death meant just leaving the stage long enough to change costume and come back as a new character ... Would you slow down? Or speed up?"

– Chuck Palahniuk

Having broadened the discussion of dual diagnosis in the last chapter and provided clinical cases to illustrate the condition, I would now like to provide some historical background to put into perspective what causes dual diagnosis. There are two theories of historical significance: Darwin's theory of natural selection and Mendel's theories of inheritance. Each complements the other.

Charles Darwin was a naturalist who studied the adaptive characteristics of various species of finches in the Galapagos Islands. His theory of natural selection, laid out in his 1859 book, *The Origin of the Species,* became the accepted mechanism by which the evolution of all species was presumed to have occurred. However, it was Gregor Mendel, now regarded as the father of modern genetics, who proposed two separate theories – The Law of Independent Assortment and the Law of Segregation – that helped to provide a foundation for Darwin's conclusions. Mendel's paper, *Experiments on Plant Hybridization*, was published in 1866.

In my opinion, it was the identification of DNA, the basis of all life on Earth, by Swiss chemist Friedrich Miescher in the 1860s that consolidated the efforts of Darwin and Mendel. Most people mistakenly assume that DNA was discovered in the mid-1950s by James Watson and Francis Crick of Cambridge University. What Watson and Crick actually did was to elucidate the chemical structure of DNA, a feat for which they received the Nobel Prize almost a century after Miescher's discovery.

Our understanding today is that DNA, or biological intelligence, is not a static entity but a dynamic one. I liken it to an air traffic control tower rather than the blueprint it was originally conceived to be. In this newer model, "time" as we conventionally understand the concept gives way to "space-time," a concept originally coined by physicist Albert Einstein, and hence biological intelligence is considered more virtual than linear. By this I mean that all biological events are posited to be occurring simultaneously within four-dimensional space, including time, such that a single molecule can literally oversee untold biological processes without having to rely upon any external intelligence.

At the level of the mind, cause and effect are also fluid, just as throwing a stone upon water creates ripples. The term "mind" refers in fact to an all-encompassing field that is localizable neither in space nor time as these entities exist in three-dimensions: it is omnipresent, which is to say that it is found anywhere and everywhere within consciousness, with the virtual intelligence of DNA serving as command center.

Using a similar analogy, I would liken a dual diagnosis to the epicenter of an earthquake: once the damage is done, it is irrevocable based on our current understanding, but, from a management perspective, if we wish to localize and confine that epicenter, we first need to have an idea where the fault lines lie. I have defined belief systems as the sum total of an individual's ideas, attitudes, beliefs and values, and I believe they are a core issue to consider.

Let me qualify the above statement by pointing out that ideas, attitudes and beliefs often vary considerably from generation to generation. Values, on the other hand, tend to be much more deeply ingrained. They represent the characteristics of a society that validate and perpetuate that specific social system, so they tend by definition to self-perpetuate until they are obsolete, and even far beyond when their shelf-life expires.

Most people would tend to ascribe a moral connotation to their values. At the risk of splitting hairs, I do not believe that is entirely correct. What then is the difference between morals and values? Morals help an individual decide between what is categorically right and wrong. Ideally, values have a pedagogical function, that of guiding the individual smoothly through the various stages of life.

Values essentially serve an adaptive function. In the case of the family unit, they are imbibed as if by osmosis, and they either can assist the individual in facing and coping with life, or they can prove disabling, in which case the individual succumbs to the life circumstances he or she has been dealt with given the values that have been modeled within the home. Which is not necessarily bleak. Take for instance the gifted artist who gives up his or her avowed true passion and ends up perpetuating the family values by going to Harvard and becoming a brilliant third-generation surgeon.

Indigenous populations of the world have a lot to teach Western society about sustainable values, though these lessons have come at a terrible price. By and large these proud peoples have been stripped of their values and native heritage, decimated by slavery or colonization and the scourge of imported illness, or plundered by the advance of industrialization and racial prejudice. It is only through the rekindling of native spiritual practices that the younger generations are now coming back into their birthright, particularly in North America.

Modern humans themselves are mired in an anguished search for self. Our society is on the cusp of profound cultural changes. People aren't buying set formulas anymore, nor the pious platitudes of eras gone by. We are prone as never before to existential angst, or so it seems, and the beaten track brings neither comfort nor hope, much less awakening. Unfortunately, both mental illness and addiction are symptomatic of this profound deficit.

Many of the diseases of so-called modern humans are both a product and a reflection of their social condition. Curiously enough, addiction was unknown to the aboriginal peoples of the Americas. But how did these cultures deal with the phenomenon of mental illness? Each tribe had its shaman, medicine man or native healer.

Shamans were individuals who, during the course of their early development, either as children or as teenagers, had had a tumultuous psychological experience that catapulted the entire psyche inward. Those who succeeded in integrating the demonic or deistic elements encountered there into their personality emerged strengthened from the experience, and equipped henceforth with deeper and visionary insights to help the tribe survive. Many were then trained by elder shamans and other keepers of the clan's wisdom or through further exploration of their inner worlds, often with the aid of sacred psychotropic drugs.

Whatever the method, shamans became adept at guiding others who were experiencing crises of the psyche to gain a firm foothold on reality, be it through native pharmacopoeia, incantation or ritual, including dream questing. In this sense, aboriginal peoples had a true understanding of mental illness as something that affects the subconscious. To me, the general practitioner (GP) plays the role of the modern-day shaman in many ways.

Western medicine has adopted the scientific method for the study and treatment of mental illness. It is hard to imagine that it still relies in part on Newtonian mechanics devised over 300 years ago. By focusing more on the chemical and mechanical aspects and ignoring the energetic dimension of reality, it limits the understanding of healing to what I consider to be a great extent. Newtonian logic and methods work for disorders that have a physical origin, such as trauma, physical deficiencies, poisonings and infections. But physical illness can also stem from energetic dimensions that are affected by one's beliefs, attitudes and thoughts, and this is often the case with dual diagnosis.

Our current bio-psychosocial model for treating dual diagnosis was first proposed by psychiatrist George Engel in 1977, and it was primarily directed at physicians and health care workers. The model I advocate is more patient-centered: it addresses the energetic component of human illness and recognizes a spiritual dimension that is core to all healing.

To me, what is needed is a model of care in which the general practitioner creates "the spoke in the wheel" so to speak. At the epicenter of this model, unaffected by outward circumstance, is the patient's innate and ever-abiding spiritual connection to a Higher Self or Divine Presence, whatever the name of choice. The primary role of the GP is to facilitate the connection between that epicenter and the outer rim of the wheel, represented by functional stability in the patient's everyday life. The sturdiness of the wheel equates to the state of the individual's general health and well-being.

I do not believe that one can actually correct or eradicate emotional, mental or spiritual problems with purely material remedies or physical manipulations. Yes, it may be possible to improve the condition for a time or to mask the symptoms and physical effects by such means. But emotional, mental and spiritual disorders *per se* need to be treated at the same or higher level than where the dysfunction originates. In this respect, spiritual solutions best resolve mental problems, and rational understanding more effectively resolves emotional problems. When a condition is treated from below the originating level, it is my experience that negative side effects, complications and unexpected relapses tend to arise.

Fortunately, many of society's ills are just the result of a lack of common sense. Our education system is primarily at fault. Some would argue that acquiring a sense of responsibility, punctuality, respect and discipline are more than adequate end goals along with basic academic proficiency in what used to be called "the 3 Rs." But what of those individuals, including many with a dual diagnosis, who fall between the cracks? Are they to be herded through with the rest of the fold only to be cast aside after high school graduation, if they even make it that far?

It is my belief that every child should be regarded as unique and given the opportunity to climb the ladder of success whether he or she is in need of specialized attention or not. Individuals can be given aptitude testing as required and then directed along the appropriate path. This is not to say that education is about summarily separating the wheat from the chaff for progressively more cutthroat stakes. Rather, it should aim to instill self-esteem, self-confidence and a winning attitude in all. Some may simply be better served by leaving the traditional school system and being educated in some alternate manner, including the very gifted.

When it comes to the dually-diagnosed, we need to identify not only which individuals have not succeeded within the traditional school system but also *why* they have not succeeded. As it was pointed out in Chapter 1, mental illness and addiction are often all but entrenched by the time a child is in his or her teens. As we saw in Chapter 2, we are often dealing with familial and societal attitudes that address only the surface of the problem. At the stage where neither overt mental illness nor addiction are present, genetic and environmental factors need to be considered and preempted or counterbalanced in some way so that an individual who is battling the odds can have a fighting chance.

Societal attitudes toward the dually diagnosed need to change such that these individuals be afforded the right to hold an esteemed position within society. Just to clarify that point, it is not the position itself but the aptitude and attitude of the individual holding the position that count, plus his or her sense of accomplishment in doing the job well. Once there is a genuine foundation for self-esteem, there will be no need for these kids to look elsewhere to validate their experience.

Whatever course of action one elects to follow in life, there seems to be a magnetic correlation between one's ability to rise to the inevitable challenges and the presence of a functional belief system that is fully integrated. Psychologists now understand that a substantial cross-section of the individual's character traits develop during the formative years, so the longer it takes to identify and confront a potential problem, the more entrenched it becomes. Some 10 or 15 years later, it is often too late to correct troublesome issues that could effectively have been nipped in the bud if identified at a much earlier stage. By the same token, something that would have been considered a minor problem if identified at the outset is far more difficult to address later in life, sometimes even to the point of being cast in stone.

In the broader arena, I would suggest that before we can overcome many of the prejudices that limit our progress as a global society, we need to re-assess some of our cherished attitudes and beliefs by examining the values that underlie them. Take materialism as an example of an explicit value system.

It is one thing to look upon the plight of the Third World and feel a deep sense of empathy for those who live there under abject circumstances, but how ready are we to acknowledge how much our Western lifestyle is directly responsible for and perpetuating that great divide? At last count, less than 20% of the world's population wastes and usurps 80% of its resources. Is there not some fundamental incongruence here?

Another random example of skewed values is how little depth or credibility many role models possess today. Name three celebrities the younger generation look up to and long to emulate. Do you think any of these people or the fads they represent are likely to be anything more that a footnote to society 50 years from now?

In another vein, the current Western stereotype of adult womanly beauty is unsustainable for all but a minuscule few. I am reminded of a quip circulating on the Internet a few years back to the effect that there are over three billion women in the world today but only seven or eight supermodels. Underlying this sad assertion is that women collectively are still being coveted today as objects of desire or valued as mere chattels – if they count at all – rather than being respected for being who they are.

Another modern-values fallacy is the prevalence of the nuclear family. This is a concept alien to most aboriginal societies and certainly to those throughout the

East, where extended and joint families are the norm. Even in the West, less than 25% of families today fit the pattern of two parents, one of either sex, sharing the duties of child rearing. It would seem as often as not, single young females are now heading up single-parent households. In sum, the so-called "traditional" family is just not the reality anymore.

I still feel that children need a stable family structure in order to develop stable, balanced personalities and best learn to deal with life on life's terms. However, traditional marriage as a social institution does not necessarily guarantee a stable family life. Once again, I stress the importance of putting into place a mature, functioning belief system. An individual who is accountable to him- or herself can then be counted on by and large to be accountable to and for others. Let's take a look at a case study.

"Zoltan" recently celebrated his eighteenth year of sobriety. He is Serbian and was born into the Eastern Orthodox faith. His mother was an alcoholic and his father was an enabler. His family life as a child was turbulent. He was raised a Christian as was "Alexis," his partner, who is also an alcoholic. The difference is that "Alexis" is a practicing Christian whereas "Zoltan" no longer attends church services. Although "Zoltan" and "Alexis" are not married, they have conceived a child together, "Jakob," who is now two years old. "Alexis" has two other children from two separate fathers but she apparently sees something in "Zoltan" that she especially cherishes. I expect that this couple have their ups and downs like most couples do, but it is clear that together they stand for something that neither is capable of generating alone. I am happy to report that both are currently sober.

He may no longer go to church, but "Zoltan" attends on average two meetings of Alcoholics Anonymous (AA) a day. He exhibits prominent bipolar traits and, truth be told, if it were not for these meetings, his life would undoubtedly fall to pieces within a short time. He would most definitely benefit from mood-stabilizing medication if only he would agree to it.

"Zoltan" is fully aware of the fact that his stability is somewhat tenuous. He knows from experience that when he is glib and does not give the meetings his full attention, his spiritual condition rapidly deteriorates. Still, "Zoltan" is by no means a social misfit and he is spiritually fit, at least for today. Though his life has been filled with struggle, to the point where he recently declared bankruptcy, "Zoltan" has determined that the load is infinitely easier to bear with AA, and has tremendous faith in the power of his meetings. In fact, he gets quite irritated if anything interferes, even his family life.

However, having interacted with baby "Jakob" on several occasions, I can attest that "Zoltan" experiences a genuine release from his conditioned thinking as a result of the meetings. The important thing is that neither he nor "Alexis" is currently using and they care deeply for one another. "Jakob" is growing and developing normally. He is an adorable, happy child and both "Alexis" and "Zoltan" dote on him.

I have chosen this case history to illustrate the importance of having a solid belief system, whatever the basis. Though "Zoltan" has broken with the Church, he is a wholesome man in many ways thanks to AA. Still, his life experience, as mentioned, has been less than ideal and his values continue somewhat to reflect this fact. The sad truth is that "Zoltan" has had to learn everything he now goes by from scratch, and he began to do so only once he entered Alcoholics Anonymous.

To me, it does not matter by what name "Zoltan" calls his Higher Power because his positive actions speak for themselves. There is, however, a caveat. Addiction is a cunning, baffling and powerful disease. Despite his 18 years of commitment to not drinking, "Zoltan" remains what would typically be considered a true alcoholic. He is "clean" in that he clings for dear life to attending his two AA meetings a day, more or less without fail. His is an example of spiritual progress, not spiritual perfection.

"Zoltan" has realized that he does have a choice; he can wallow in self-pity or he can take a stand. But abstinence is not recovery. It is relationships that form the cornerstone of recovery from both mood-altering substance abuse and mental illness. At the heart of "Zoltan's" unresolved condition are fear and a deep-seated sense of insecurity. I contend that these traits are both a reflection and a product of childhood trauma that no amount of faith can remove, at least not in "Zoltan's" case.

The more deep-seated the insecurity, the stronger the attachment to an answer that brings temporary relief. So although AA has apparently effected a radical transformation in "Zoltan," especially when viewed in hindsight, in truth its influence can be considered a moderating one at best because "Zoltan" is still not whole. He suffers from psychological dependency as well as his bipolar issues.

If more self-knowledge could be counted on to bring about the ultimate resolution of "Zoltan's" ills, how far would I say he is from experiencing his true self? Well, before this can happen, I suggest that he needs to transcend his ego or the image he has created of himself. To his credit, he has travelled somewhat along the path by giving freely of himself in service to other AA members.

Through AA, "Zoltan" has come to appreciate the value of basic life skills and tools such as discipline and accountability for one's actions. Undoubtedly, the fellowship has also taught him the value of humility and opened the door for him to a deeper experience of the human condition. However, what "Zoltan" still fundamentally lacks is self-control. In many respects, he is an accident waiting to happen. Each time I see him in the office, he is transiting in and out of crisis. His life is melodramatic to say the least, and in a strange sort of way, he seems to thrive on the excitement. Perhaps chaos is what he knows best. Certainly, the insanity in his life is mostly of his own making.

Like "Zoltan," most members of self-help fellowships move through the Harm Reduction paradigm whereby substance abuse is either gradually tapered through consecutive phases of medical management, or they completely abstain with varying levels of success. We will discuss the philosophy of Harm Reduction at greater length later. As far as the mental illness component of a dual diagnosis goes, compliance with the medication guidelines inevitably remains a major component affecting the patient's overall outcome.

In my opinion, though self-help fellowships are useful, they can often merely replace one form of dependency with another. "Zoltan" is just as addicted to his AA meetings as he was to his drug of choice when he was actively using. His life is arguably better, but his stability remains tenuous.

Some may argue that belief in a Higher Power is not a dependency in the regular sense of the word. I beg to differ. In my view what is all-important is faith, which I define as a *reliance* on God, not a dependence. Reliance encompasses the term self-reliance which is based upon the broader notion of self-knowledge used within Eastern parlance, and reinforces the point that in order for real change to occur, one must be willing to do at least some of the work. Real power comes from within, and true understanding implies action.

One overriding criticism of self-help fellowships is that they don't work. Well, that is perhaps a bit harsh. I would just say that there is a general lack of hard statistical evidence or other scientific proof to outweigh the by-in-large anecdotal evidence that these programs are effective. In support of the criticism, however, I have met many alcoholics in the AA program who fell off the wagon after many years of consecutive sobriety and ended up leaving a path of devastation in their wake.

What are the values we should be honoring within Canadian society? First and foremost any value system adopted must be sustainable. Social democratic thought has inspired legislation to entrench such benefits as worker's compensation, minimum wage, old-age pension, unemployment insurance, family allowance, subsidized housing and medicare. The welfare state has largely been the product of joint action by new democrats and reform-minded liberals based on a belief that capitalism and democratic rights can coexist in such a way that all segments of society benefit. In recent years, however, social democratic doctrine has come under increasing criticism from both left- and right-wing elements.

The radical and revolutionary Left charges that social democratic reforms are too eclectic, targeting too few and mostly unprofitable industries. They cite detailed analyses to prove that the welfare state has not altered class inequality to the degree expected and that poverty in Canada is more firmly rooted than ever. In sum, social democracy to them has produced only cosmetic changes at best, making capitalism appear more humane and workable, and delaying needed structural changes.

By definition, the goal of the Far Left is socialism, not social democracy. The problem is that the word itself almost universally raises the specter of communism, its dreaded-though-more-or-less-defunct brother. Not very many people in this country have any meaningful conception of what "socialism" might entail as a workable political platform.

The welfare state is also under attack by right-wing neo-conservatives critical of large increases in government expenditure and the size of the civil service. They note that economic growth is now slowing down and that the combination of high unemployment and higher inflation rates not only confirms the menace of reduced productivity, but is the harbinger of funds running out with which to finance social spending. One result is that programs such as universal medicare are being ever more stridently attacked by this faction. This is obviously a concern to someone like me who works closely with a number of marginalized elements within the community including the dually-diagnosed.

How has this clash of political extremes and all of the ensuing political rhetoric affected societal attitudes? Well, instead of the social foment one might expect the battle of ideologies to generate in the body politic, there has instead been an increase in apathy as evidenced by poor voter turnout and a lack of public participation at the municipal and regional levels.

And how much of this vacuum can we attribute to a general absence of media focus on reporting changes in public policy, both contemplated and implemented, so that all sectors of the public know what is going on? Instead of fulfilling a key role as watchdogs in defense of the public good, the radio and television industries have increasingly and rather consistently been morphing into straight-line purveyors of entertainment.

In my opinion, North American society is eroding from a cultural point of view and this is evidenced primarily by a lack of clear-cut identity. We seem to be constantly striving to reinvent ourselves, but the concept is so fractured and fuzzy that we are missing the boat entirely. We just do not know who we are anymore. Our institutions, our ideals and our role models all lack even the most basic credibility, with the inevitable result that as a society, we are floundering for even a whiff of the correct direction in which to move.

I further submit that our society has become a breeding ground for illnesses such as lung cancer, obesity, diabetes and heart disease that are predominantly the result of self-defeating lifestyle choices. An estimated 85% of chronic illnesses are attributable to our diet and the ways in which we choose to live and think. These choices in turn are largely due to an almost pathological preoccupation on our part with immediate gratification. As a result, consumerism now reigns supreme, to the detriment of the tried and true values that upheld society until not so long ago. I sometimes wonder if we aren't suffering from some form of collective Narcissistic Personality Disorder!

In my own sphere of expertise, I contend that the prevalence of dual diagnosis in Canada has been grossly underestimated due to sampling error. Were a large enough population to be surveyed, and were the sample correctly weighted as concerns age, gender and socioeconomic variables, I feel confident in surmising that dual diagnosis affects about 25% to 30% of the adult population, both in Canada and in North America overall (as a conservative estimate). If one takes into account that we are talking about a chronically relapsing and remitting condition, estimates may range even higher. I would now like to digress slightly and elaborate upon this particular point.

A review of the literature on dual diagnosis reveals discrepant findings for many of the conditions being reported. Some of the problems plaguing the studies reviewed attempting to document prevalence rates for dual diagnosis include a basic failure to correlate study design and methodology in their analysis. The net result is that what is being reported is not an accurate reflection of what the researchers are attempting to measure. Consequently, discrepant findings are the norm rather than the exception within this emerging area.

Two large well-designed and methodologically-sound longitudinal studies done in community-based settings – the Epidemiologic Catchment Area Study

(ECA) and the National Comorbidity Survey (NCS) done in the US – have established the heterogeneity of psychiatric disorders in substance abusing patients in general. [1, 2] Both the ECA study and NCS have established that the lifetime prevalence risk of developing a comorbid psychiatric disorder subsequent to having an established SUD exceeds the risk within the general population by an estimated 2 to 3 times. A recent meta-analysis (a pooling of results reported over a number of different studies) has shown that within opiod-dependent patients psychiatric comorbidity occurs at the following rates: 78.3% with at least one co-occurring psychiatric disorder, 42.2% with a personality disorder, 31.2% with a mood disorder and 8% with an anxiety disorder [3].

The real solution for Canada is to reexamine our priorities as a nation. In particular, our social agenda and the values we should be nurturing in the younger generation need to become a focus of debate in Parliament. One fundamental question we should be asking is whether pure capitalism, at least as it now functions, is not at odds with our social agenda.

Our friends south of the border have witnessed a fight to the death pitting the privileged Old Guard against President Obama's proposed health care reforms. Our health care system is one of Canada's most unique assets and an inspiration to less fortunate parts of the world and countries where social disparity is still rampant, including the US. It behooves us to remember and safeguard our precious legacy.

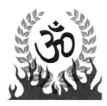

CHAPTER 4

NARCISSISTIC PERSONALITY DISORDER

"My brain: it's my second favorite organ."

– Woody Allen

The personality disorders described throughout this work comprise a heterogeneous group, or a "mixed bag" in lay terms. Collectively, they have baffled attempts to elucidate their causes and origins and to devise the best treatments, which by and large currently involve some form of intensive psychotherapy. When it comes to their association within the framework of a dual diagnosis, four so-called Cluster B personality disorders are most characteristically associated with a substance use disorder.

Although the conditions are considered rare in a sampling of the general populace, within my practice I see the Cluster B personality disorders fairly often, and Narcissistic Personality Disorder in particular. Borderline Personality Disorder, Sociopathic Personality Disorder and, less commonly, Histrionic Personality Disorder follow in that order. Most sociopaths are male whereas the other three disorders tend to occur more commonly in females.

Having worked with a number of disordered personalities and also having achieved some success in meeting short-term and intermediate objectives during the course of managing these individuals, I would say that my main objective has been to facilitate the development of a stable core in my patients. These individuals respond best to discipline and the need to be accountable and rigorously honest.

The initial assessment develops over several visits where an attempt is made to identify the core issues that the individual is grappling with such as control, trust, dependency and so forth. Classic examples are provided throughout this book that show how these core issues manifest and how they are best dealt with. When the assessment has been completed, a strategy is put into place whereby the patient is incrementally challenged to meet and ultimately surpass a set of short-term objectives. This process is staggered so that progress can be seen to occur, at least in retrospect.

Let's now take a look at "Sean," our case study for this chapter. He is the product of a teen pregnancy complicated by substance abuse. Both his parents were alcoholics but are now sober. His father has recently been diagnosed as HIV+. Having experienced a fair amount of childhood trauma, "Sean" dropped out of school at a young age and has been on his own from the age of 15. Though not formally educated, he is street smart.

"Sean" decided to go back to school after fifteen years to get a diploma in licensed practical nursing. It was then that he began having panic attacks and came to see me. "Sean" exhibited a background of self-deprecating thoughts, self-limiting beliefs and marked perfectionism. Oddly enough, he also manifested a tendency toward self-sabotage during our encounters. Unfortunately, his self-destructive behavior did not stop there. After a few sessions, "Sean" informed me that when his thinking became too much of a nuisance or when his anxiety level was intolerable, he would binge drink. Needless to say, he was failing at least one course at career college.

The more I got to know "Sean," the more I realized how tightly wound he was. Ultimately, I diagnosed him with Obsessive Compulsive Disorder in addition to a substance use disorder. With the help of counseling and fairly lofty doses of medication, he overcame the OCD, at least functionally, and his substance abuse gradually tapered once this mental illness was appropriately medicated.

The curious thing in "Sean's" case, at least to me, was that all of his problems seemed to stem from his religious upbringing. His belief system was more or less a childhood fantasy that he never outgrew. To me, this suggested a history of childhood trauma, and as I got to know "Sean" more, he confirmed my suspicions in this regard.

Beliefs are powerful! When they can no longer be contained within the narrow boundaries of an antiquated and overtaxed system, people often suffer what is commonly called a "nervous breakdown." The ego feels threatened as the person begins to fall apart, and it intensifies the basic survival instinct. Un-checked, this intensification causes anxiety, obsessive thinking, compulsions (as was borne out in this case) and, at the far end of the spectrum, psychotic symptoms. The chemical imbalance within the brain is often compounded by the use of mood-altering substances.

"Sean" had difficulty accepting the diagnosis of OCD. In fact, most of the session in which I informed him of my clinical suspicions consisted of him telling me all the reasons why he thought my diagnosis was wrong. Nonethe-less, I stood firm and during the next session, he did an about-face. Initially, I found this puzzling, but his behaviors began to make sense once I realized that he was also struggling with control issues.

Some months down the road, all "Sean's" thrashing about concerning his diagnosis dissipated and something quite curious happened. His deeper consciousness, which all the while had remained submerged, awakened. The result was a noticeable reduction in his anxiety level. Rather than struggling to disengage from his diagnosis, which only served to perpetuate his wrestling to gain the upper hand, "Sean" finally surrendered. That acceptance opened the door for him to a greater reality.

"Sean" originally came to see me because he was having a difficult time dealing with the breakup with his ex-girlfriend. In fact, he was on the verge of a nervous breakdown over that. The last time we met, he informed me that school was a very lonely place for him and that he had begun dating again. "Sean" could have simply admitted he wanted an emotional connection in his life and left it at that, but it was almost as if he derived a special pleasure from informing me that he was sleeping with his present partner.

When I asked him whether he wished to get tested for sexually transmitted diseases, he said no, he was not seriously interested in his current liaison. Not only was he entirely focused on meeting his own needs, but he was also loath to admit there was anything wrong with this attitude. I began to wonder if he was not suffering from Narcissistic Personality Disorder.

As mentioned earlier, Narcissistic Personality Disorder (NPD) is one of four Cluster B personality disorders characteristically associated with substance abuse. The hallmark of a person afflicted with it is that, engrossed in his own world, he directs love to second-hand, shadow-like impressions he forms of others as a reflection of his own unresolved child-like needs for attention and ultimately acceptance, and is hence incapable of expressing true, reciprocal love. In the vernacular, "It's all about me, always."

The reality of "Sean's" situation is that his childhood and adolescent experiences have adversely influenced his development. His father was a Jehovah's Witness and his mother a Roman Catholic, but despite all the religion, his home life was very turbulent. At age 15, he was shown the door and walked out of his parents' life for good. To this day, with only his life experience to guide him, "Sean" struggles with who he is. Admittedly, his experience to date has not been much help to him in developing a strong and stable belief system. Still, while he no longer believes in God, he does wish to cultivate a relationship with a Higher Power. Unfortunately, true love remains an ideal rather than a reality in his life.

"Sean" has a lot of spiritual growing up to do to make up for the shortfalls in his character and in all fairness to him, his life. At this stage, I would say that he is at least narcissistically inclined. What I mean by that is that he has his own best interest at heart most if not all of the time. Not surprisingly, he is still somewhat dependent on others to meet his needs. What is more, he has several other core issues to come to terms with. Chief among them is trust, and he needs to work on erecting and maintaining meaningful boundaries. Hopefully, with the appropriate therapy and guidance, "Sean" will grow up, and as he does, become able to meet others on common ground. For now, he remains deeply wounded.

I find it intriguing that "Sean" should say that what he most desires is to cultivate a relationship with a Higher Power. At this point, his worst enemy is his mind, though he does intuitively understand that a higher reality is accessed through an inner, contemplative doorway rather than a cognitive one. In all fairness to him, "Sean" has learned from bitter experience that life is, on one very important level, a game of survival. He does understand, however, that there are other dimensions.

As I mentioned, I do not think "Sean" has a true Narcissistic Personality Disorder. Still, the narcissistic manner of perceiving and relating to his environment colors his relationships and always ends up causing havoc over time. Due to his dependency, he is also quite insecure, which gives others, like his choice of girlfriends, an edge upon which to prey. At age 38, "Sean" has had his first true awakening in coming to terms with his OCD. Realizing at this point that he was in fact capable of expressing genuine emotion with the former girlfriend must have been somewhat of a revelation to him.

What predisposes an individual like "Sean" or others we have studied so far in this book to a dual diagnosis? Well, attempting to integrate what I have said thus far, I would say that more often than not in the dually-diagnosed, it is the lack of a solid sense of "self," coupled with a lack of proficiency in erecting and maintaining healthy personal boundaries. One must know who one is, but also who one is not.

I have discussed the concept of boundaries in some detail in chapter 2. What I wish to add here is that those who do not have at least an intuitive sense of who they are remain incapable of knowing, protecting and truly enjoying the real self. These difficulties manifest most clearly within the complexities of human relationships. Not knowing themselves, they end up with the wrong person. Not knowing how to protect themselves, they fall prey to their circumstances in life. Not knowing how to enjoy life, they end up searching, ever unrealized, in all the wrong places. A fundamental question for such people to eventually face is "Who am I?"

Awareness begins with the process of witnessing. But witnessing, by its very nature, describes a relationship that entails both subject and object, a relationship where the ego is present, engaged in the act. So it is a preliminary stage, a means of reaching for awareness.

Awareness itself is a total, integrated state, completely devoid of such concepts as subjectivity and objectivity. There is no one who is witnessing in awareness; there is no one who is being witnessed. The subject and the object are not related in awareness, they are dissolved.

There is a wonderful walking meditation that comes from the Southern Theravada Buddhist school, the point of which is to become fully present in the "now." It goes something like this:

There is the movement of the foot. There is the perception of the feeling of the movement of the foot. There is the tendency toward the perception of the feeling of the movement of the foot. There is the consciousness of the tendency toward the perception of the feeling of the movement of the foot.

Yoga is another popular path to awareness. The name itself comes from the Sanskrit root *yuj* which means "to yoke" – to connect or join something to something else. What is being yoked is self-consciousness and the very source of consciousness, which is pure presence. In the last century or so, yoga has become an increasingly popular pastime amongst people in the West seeking union with the Divine in some aspect or form. On occasion, I have used the principles of yoga to facilitate spiritual clarity in my clients, and in some cases, with astonishing success. Many are thrilled at how much their lives have changed for the better.

Like any discipline, yoga takes practice. One of its main purposes is to quiet the mind and instruct it to function in the way it was originally intended to do, so that one's original wholeness can be accessed. Awareness is achieved initially by focusing the energies of the mind through concentration and then, at a later stage, by learning to relax the mind while it is actively concentrating. Quiet, watchful attention is the mother of true intelligence.

It is no surprise that yoga has had an esteemed position within Indian culture since its inception millennia ago. To me as a longtime practitioner, its appeal stems from the fact that it amalgamates self-knowledge and faith into a spiritual discipline that facilitates greater awareness. The fundamental goal of all three components remains nonetheless the same – to come to an awareness of who one is.

Allow me to introduce at this point two key concepts of yoga: kundalini fire and what is known in the East as the "chakras." I will very briefly explain these terms because I want to show how they relate to some of the psychospiritual elements we have been discussing up to now in Western parlance.

The word "chakra" means "wheel of light" or "spinning wheel of energy" in Sanskrit. There are seven major chakras or energy centers vertically aligned in the center of the body close to and roughly following the spine. We cannot see them since they function at the etheric level, but they serve as valves to circulate and regulate the flow of energy, the life force, throughout the body, and each has a particular significance and function.

The first chakra, known as the root chakra, is located at the base of the spine. It is said to be the seat of our procreative, survival and base instincts. The second chakra is known as the sacral chakra and it is located in the genital area. It will come as no surprise that what we have so far called the ego is rooted in these two chakras. As we have already discussed, the ego constitutes our survival instinct, and its primary objective is to indulge its voracious appetite for experience at every conceivable opportunity.

The mastery of the baser instincts and the emotions is symbolized by the control of the third or solar plexus chakra, located at stomach level just below the diaphragm. When it is not balanced, rampant "ego inflation" can occur. This is a term originally coined by C.J. Jung to describe the phenomenon whereby one perceives that outside forces are simultaneously under the control of one's own will, as in being able to fly or leap unharmed from tall buildings.

The phenomenon is somewhat analogous to the older term, "oceanism," coined by Sigmund Freud. Here the individual experiences a sensation of unbounded oneness with the universe. Both ego inflation and the oceanic phenomenon are pre-personal experiences, suggesting a collapse of definable boundaries.

Let me here interject a word about *kundalini*. It is defined as the energy that subtends the life force, and in most people, it lies dormant within the pelvis and coiled like a snake. If and when awakened, it rises from the base of the spine, at the level of the first chakra or spiritual center, and moves progressively upward, piercing the subsequent centers until it reaches the seventh or crown chakra at the top of the head, where it freely enters and exits the body.

There is a branch of yoga called kundalini yoga or the yoga of awareness, which aims to awaken the kundalini, to raise the kundalini fire such that it pierces each center of consciousness or chakra, flooding it with progressively more subtle awareness. When the energy comes to rest at or above the fourth or heart chakra, there is a profound awakening within the individual accompanied by a general feeling of well-being that often manifests as an outpouring of emotion.

The fourth chakra marks a clearinghouse for the energy of awareness. As has been mentioned, when the kundalini fire falls below the heart chakra to the more primal centers and chakras, the individual may become susceptible to an inflated ego, rampant sexual desire and many other ills and imbalances.

At or above the fourth chakra, the kundalini fire transcends all previously entrenched, self-imposed limitations. One comes to an awareness that "I Am" is a very provocative statement. Certainly, each of us is innately more than a mass of contradictory impulses and desires. In fact, in yogic terms, at precisely the point where one realizes the implicit truth of the "I Am," the fifth or throat chakra, the centre of creativity and expressiveness, symbolically crystallizes.

The sixth chakra, located between the eyebrows and sometimes called the Third Eye, is the directing center for the individual. It relates to purposeful awareness as this applies to being responsible for one's own needs and finding one's spiritual path. It also strengthens the imagination and the intuition needed to guide our lives and provides access to psychic powers.

The seventh chakra, also called the crown chakra, represents the joining of individual consciousness and the source of consciousness. When this occurs, all limitations are transcended and the "I Am" is dissolved. On the surface, this appears to be a contradiction. What is implied, however, is not the absence of boundaries but their relaxation. In Christian terms, it is an experience of the Christ Consciousness or Divine Presence within us all. Once that core identity has been experienced and realized, it remains intact regardless of any outward circumstance that may befall us.

There is a complete and very profound science of the chakras that I invite you to explore if you are so inclined, especially as it concerns alternative health and healing. As we have already mentioned, Kundalini forms a complete branch of yoga on its own that is sometimes called the yoga of awareness.

Kundalini is also sometimes referred to as the union of shakti and shiva. Shakti is defined by the dictionary as "the vital generative and creative principle at work in the universe, typically associated with the feminine component of the Divine." It is often embodied as a goddess of that name, and worshipped as the consort of the Lord Shiva.

Lord Shiva himself, sometimes termed the Destroyer, is often portrayed as the Nataraja or Lord of the Dance. In this form, he is seen dancing within an eternal ring of flames. His upper right hand holds a small drum for beating out rhythm, and his upper left, a devouring flame symbolizing change. His lower right hand is raised in the "fear not" gesture, although the arm carries a cobra, while his left arm points to a foot lifted to symbolize "release." The other foot is planted on the squirming body of the demon of ignorance and heedlessness. The Nataraja figure dramatizes the vital processes of the universe, bringing together the themes of death and rebirth.

CHAPTER 5

BORDERLINE PERSONALITY DISORDER

"I used to be Snow White, but I drifted."

– Mae West

Historically, Western society has been influenced by two predominant myths or images that are used to make sense of reality. The first, which has been termed the "ceramic model," posits that man was made in God's image much like a clay pot is molded by a potter. The problem with this idea is that man is not fabricated in the same way as a clay pot. All life grows and, in so doing, progressively complicates itself.

This first myth traces its origins to the *Book of Genesis* where God purportedly created the Earth and the heavens in six days and rested on the seventh. It dominated right up to the Renaissance, when scientific achievements and theories of the cosmos such as the heliocentrism of Nicolaus Copernicus began to overshadow it.

The second myth has been called the "fully automatic model" of the universe and it began to take shape as a result of such theories. Gaining popularity over the centuries, the essential premise of this model is that the universe is one big wind-up toy created for mankind's amusement. It appeals in that it downplays the role of God as central to the cosmic machine, and substitutes humankind as the protagonist. Secondarily, it enthrones the scientific hypothesis and the power of scientific prediction as determinants of reality as we know it. Newton's laws of motion and Freud's theory of libido or blind lust are directly attributable to it.

As a matter of some curiosity, even the colonization of the New World could be deemed a direct descendant, the idea being that in line with this model, humankind is just a "fluke" of the universe and that it must do constant battle to assert supremacy over Mother Nature. That said, various scientific theories have emerged either to support or refute this contention.

Let me digress ever so slightly here to open a new topic that will ultimately tie back to the two models under discussion. The human brain is a remarkable organ, consisting of billions upon billions of nerve cells dying and being replaced every day in their legions, while the organ itself, for most of us, remains coherent throughout our lifespan. There are two radically opposed accounts, however, of what the function of the brain is. The first and most familiar is entirely in keeping with our second myth. It posits that the brain is a thought generator and that its ability to function as such has developed incrementally and accidentally over billions of years in the manner described in Charles Darwin's *On the Origin of Species*.

The other more radical account, which is gradually overtaking its predecessor, is perhaps most effectively presented in the work of Rudolf Steiner. [1] He insisted that the brain's primary function is not to be a generator of thought but rather an organ of perception, and his proposition is finding new support in quantum physics.

Experiments performed in the 1940s by the eminent Canadian neurosurgeon Wilder Penfield revealed that the brain is the *recorder* of experience whereas the mind is the *generator* of experience. Penfield's conclusions led to the proposition that the mind is in fact a quantum field, and the brain is simply an organ where thought is linguistically structured. Thought as such is a "space-time" or quantum event, and it occurs anywhere and everywhere within consciousness.

It follows then that whatever truth lies within our little corner of the galaxy is symptomatic of the entire company of galaxies dancing in procession one with another. "As above, so below," and mankind serves as an aperture by which the entire universe is exploring itself. Science itself is beginning to posit that some form of Creative Intelligence – whatever the name ascribed to it – underpins the entire workings of the universe.

Accordingly, a new myth has begun to emerge whose origins can be traced to developments in theoretical physics in the early part of the 20th century. In part, it surmises that evolution is a random walk in space-time, at least as concerns the individual. But it is also toying with the notion that the universe is a compassionate one and that the odds are stacked in our favor right from the start. Universal Intelligence as yet cannot be fully comprehended, but the search is on for the basic "stuff" that constitutes all matter. Some have called this entity Quantum Gravity. In line with this new myth, the individual's real identity is said to be one with the source of all consciousness.

There are two ways to direct the discussion at this point! One is to compare and contrast the notion of consciousness as viewed in the East and in the West, and the other is to explore some Eastern creation myths in line with the ones we have presented so far. Let us start with elements of consciousness.

Within the chakra system outlined in the previous chapter, experience is said to form the backbone of all acquired wisdom. However, in clinical parlance, being overly greedy for experience reflects a lack of self-regulation over the desires of the ego. As it turns out in the actual arena of life, one or many experiences can occur that have the potential to transform one's entire consciousness. The hope is that such "peak experiences" lead ultimately to the awakening of that which had always been present but has hitherto remained dormant deep within.

That "awakening" of consciousness begins with an unmasking of the delusion that one cannot be anything other than a separate self, and that this world is nothing other than what it appears to be. In reality, we are all connected to one another and to everything around us. It is man and not God who alienates himself, and in so doing, denies his true nature, which is to be one with God.

Sigmund Freud, the grandfather of psychoanalytic therapy, envisioned a fundamental schism in humankind when he conceptualized the psychodynamics of the human psyche. According to Freud's model, the *id* represents the carnal instincts of man; the *ego* is his "persona" or the mask he presents to the external world; the *superego* is the repository of his ideals. In line with mythology predominant in the West, the eternal struggle between "good" and "evil" is represented as the subconscious conflict between id and superego, leading to neurosis in the manifest ego.

The Hindu idea differs considerably in that although it recognizes the existence of an individuated self, that self is considered to be a manifestation of the Great Self. This model not only affords us a clarification of the relationship between God and man, but leads to a reconciliation between the two, opening the door to further psychological development and higher states of consciousness.

Hinduism also recognizes an awakening from delusion, this awakening is termed "moksha" or liberation. In a related notion – called "lila" in the East or the Divine Comedy in the West – the Great Self or Godhead is perceived to be acting for no explicit purpose other than its own entertainment and amusement through cycle upon cycle of complete self-absorption with the manifest world. The Supreme is said to dream up creation in all its manifest universes, and all of our so-called reality is thus but a field of illusion or "maya."

In a somewhat similar vein, it seems to me that Western society today has become mired in a net of abstractions of its own, another form of "maya," due to the erosion of its values. I would go so far as to say it is in meltdown due to abject materialism, which is being aided and abetted by the popular media and the lack of a cohesive system of education.

Curiously enough, Indian society weathered a similar experience around 600 to 500 BCE, at which time both Jain and Buddhist elements within that society broke rank and established themselves as distinct from Upanishadic or classical Hinduism. This was to be expected because Hinduism had by then diversified into so many conflicting directions that its central message had become rather dilute.

Fundamentally, neither Jainism nor Buddhism concedes the preeminence of a supraindividual Self or God. This shift in focus paved the way for secularism to flourish in Indian society. Buddhism further distinguished itself from its historical predecessor, Jainism, when the Buddha laid out his version of *dharma* or the "truth" implicit in all existence.

The original doctrine of the Buddha was atheistic, not so much because the Buddha himself had no inclination toward spiritual values, which he did, but because society at that time needed to see clear of the "God idea" in order to find its own path toward creative expression. Though it has evolved over the centuries into a major world religion, Buddhism began as a system of education, a humanitarian philosophy whose primary focus is the preservation of human values. However, the Buddhist understanding of "values" differs considerably from that of its Christian counterpart.

Let me illustrate with the Zen Buddhist story of a samurai warrior who went out one day in search of the bandit who had assassinated his overlord. Having cornered the murderer, the samurai drew his sword and was about to strike a fatal retaliatory blow. In terror, the bandit spat in his face, upon which the samurai sheathed his sword, turned and walked away.

To us in the West, this would seem an act of forgiveness, or even one of simple morality: "Thou shalt not kill." Buddhism, a composite of the values of tolerance, generosity and understanding, would view this as an act of compassion: the bandit, whatever his misdeeds, remained a sentient being. Hinduism would call the pull-back *ahimsa* or harmlessness, based on its core value to not incur bad karma. To solidify the point being made, compassion at least within Buddhist circles is a universal and not a personal act.

To return to the notion of the Supreme at play, and to continue our foray into Eastern creation myths, Hindu mythology posits that there are many world cycles and saviors. The tenth avatar or incarnation of the god Vishnu – an aspect of the Hindu godhead personifying the preservation of values – is awaited as the messiah, Kalki. It is said that he will come, with a sword of flame and riding a white horse, to save the righteous and destroy the wicked at the end of the current *yuga* or world period. To some, the horse is so prominent that they call this savior the Ashvatara or "Horse Avatar."

Kalki literally means "of iron" or machine. The world is currently in the fourth world period, known in India as the *kali yuga*. During this era, evil is said to prevail and worsen to a lowest point before order is once again established with the coming of the savior. As mentioned, the Hindu notion of time is vast and cyclical, such that when the kali yuga ends, the grand cycle of time will again repeat itself.

Adding some Western perspective, the age of Kalki, the machine age, could be said to have begun with the industrial revolution at about the turn of the 19th century. The electronic or computer age that birthed almost a century later at the midpoint of the 20th century during World War II has given humankind the ability to forge its own flaming sword, and with this new-found power has begun the tenth Ashvatara. To me, the white horse symbolizes hope for all mankind.

Let us now return to the many faces of dual diagnosis, and take a look at "Sabita" bringing the foregoing discussion into a more mundane clinical context, and reestablishing the relationship between dual diagnosis and psychospirituality. I shall now discuss another one of the cluster B personality disorders that are typically associated with a substance use disorder in the context of dual diagnosis. "Sabita" recounts:

I thought it was gonna be clear sailing all the way, but last year was the toughest year of my recovery so far. After living six months clean, I went out and binged one night, and then after another month clean, went out one more time, which led to a complete meltdown. I was "this close" to landing in jail or a mental institution. It's taken me a while to realize I can't do this thing on my own. Trying to control my using myself is just too risky.

"Sabita's" struggle with the issue of control brings to the foreground the much larger issue of her dependency. Sadly, it often takes a crisis before some headway in treating a dual diagnosis can occur. "Sabita" has what is medically termed a borderline personality and, as she herself states, she is also chemically dependent.

To those unfamiliar with the term, a person with Borderline Personality Disorder (BPD) often experiences a repetitive pattern of disorganization and instability in self-image, mood, behavior and close personal relationships. It is a common disorder, affecting as much as 10% to 14% of the general population. The frequency in women is two or three times greater than in men.

People with this disorder are often bright and can appear warm, friendly and competent. They can sometimes maintain the facade for a number of years until something happens and their defense structure crumbles. This is sometimes a stressful situation like the breakup of a romantic relationship or the death of a parent. Goals of treatment include increased self-awareness with greater impulse control and increased stability in personal relationships. A positive result would be increased tolerance of anxiety.

The diagnosis of BPD and indeed all personality disorders requires careful observation over time and over a number of situations, so it might prove illuminating to reiterate the process by which this diagnosis was established in "Sabita's" case. Having observed her on several occasions, I would repeatedly hear "Sabita" accusing her partner (also present) of wanting to leave her. At other times, she would state that she felt totally unworthy of being with him and at other times still, she would brutalize him for controlling her and keeping her away from other people.

Because of their intense fear of abandonment, borderlines have extreme and illogical sensitivities that the tiniest thing can trigger. They often fly into a rage. They can sometimes also respond by becoming despondent. At other times, they may react like narcissists, doing anything to erase a suggestion that they themselves might be flawed. In terms of their pronounced mood swings, borderlines can move through cycles lasting several days or even weeks that include periods of despondency, anger and calm. Having established that such a pattern existed in "Sabita," I became quite convinced that the diagnosis of BPD was indeed correct.

When "Sabita" is behaving appropriately, her thinking is in check. But the sense of accountability and discipline that she is fundamentally lacking needs to become entrenched so that the problems she has with impulse control and self-regulation can be mediated and overcome. I contend that when she begins to treat her chemical dependency in a big way, everything else will fall into place. What she most requires is Good Orderly Direction (GOD) to bring some measure of stability to her life.

The fundamental psychodynamic considerations in those with BPD are parental separation during childhood and a poor mother-child relationship. These facts are borne out in "Sabita's" case history. Her parents separated when she was a teenager. "Sabita" describes her mother as both powerful and distant, and states that she was not an ideal role model. From what I could gather, there seems to have been a lot of psychological abuse directed at her in childhood.

"Sabita" is part English Canadian, part East Indian. In recent years, she has re-kindled her relationship with her father, who is a practicing Hindu, and through this has begun to explore her native culture. Fortunately, AA's mission statement about believing in a Higher Power of one's own understanding has not been a problem for her. In fact, it has created the necessary space in "Sabita's" life for her to realize she is entitled to her own spiritual beliefs.

"Sabita" is also a part-time university student majoring in political science. She is quite obviously intellectually driven. The problem of simply being herself she shares to some extent with many people on the path to self-realization. The dichotomy in her case is exacerbated by her mixed Anglo-Indian heritage. By the same token, AA is classically a philosophy of Harm Reduction in practice, but in "Sabita's" case, the program is being taken to its next level – that of spiritual awakening.

When I last bumped into "Sabita," she told me she remains abstinent from all mood-altering substances and has re-connected in a big way with her East Indian culture, where she finds both peace and stability. I think that how "Sabita's" case has worked out to date is a good example of how an individual's beliefs affect the quality of his or her life. It would seem she has become enraptured with her cultural heritage and through this, I hope, she will find the direction she needs to foster tangible growth in her life.

"Sabita's" dependency is a reflection of the somewhat dysfunctional personality that was entrenched in her at a fairly young age. Substance abuse became an outlet for her frustration and aggression, confusing issues for a time and blurring her sense of identity even more. Her core issue of dependency also preempted the development of natural boundaries that would have protected the basic integrity of the self and left her unscathed.

In the absence of appropriate boundary-setting in the home, "Sabita" was unable to internalize the practices most children acquire naturally through appropriate mirroring from parental figures. Consequently, she had little if any idea of who she was as an individual, and she manufactured a fictitious image of herself. That, plus continually striving to meet the unrealistic demands placed upon her during childhood manifested the instability in her personality.

"Sabita" was conceived illegitimately and her parents then married as it seemed like the right thing to do at the time. With hindsight, they both felt otherwise. Unfortunately, "Sabita" bore the brunt of this realization. In time, she grew to understand that her mother suffered tremendously throughout the marriage. "Sabita's" family lived in a joint household with her father's family, which obviously placed an enormous further strain on her parents' relationship.

Having worked for a number of years in the Indo-Canadian community, I have observed the near-complete subjugation of individual expression to the larger cultural identity to be almost universal. This was almost assuredly a major cause of "Sabita's" mother's emotional problems, and it contributed in all likelihood to her own mental health issues as well.

In "Sabita's" case, many issues remain unresolved regarding her sense of identity. I have termed this phenomenon dependency but I now wish to clarify it as being psychological dependency. This brings me to a pivotal function of myth – the pedagogical – that of guiding the individual through the various transitions in life.

Proper child rearing ideally creates in the child a natural respect for authority. When these practices are augmented with age-appropriate values which are learned within the home, the child grows normally and during the course of natural development the individual's character is formed. When and how a functioning belief system is integrated into an individual's character to a large extent depends upon early childhood and subsequent developmental experiences which either reinforce or refute what has already been imprinted. The stability of an individual's character – meaning their ability to adapt to new and challenging situations – by-in-large is the main determinant and driver for the formation of subsequent beliefs.

Spirituality, as I use the term, is the life long process which aids in counterbalancing any perceived shortfalls in character development whereby the individual learns to process and integrate all of their experiences and hence attain ownership of them. With ownership comes responsibility and with the recognition of responsibility the potential for as-yet unrecognized growth. The main function of this growth is that it confers stability to the psyche.

Stability is to be contrasted with an adaptive advantage. The ego which is in reality only a small part of the fully developed psyche has been evolutionarily conditioned and its instincts are anticipatory and essentially fear-based. Stability calls into play an entirely different hierarchy of values coined by developmental psychologist Abraham Maslow in his 1943 paper "A Theory of Human Motivation" [2]. Here uncertainty is recognized as merely being par for the course. In this way, the element of fear is curtailed and attachment obviated because uncertainty in life can be tolerated and even embraced. An individual who is stable is one who has transcended the compulsion to control their external environment and instead has mastered self-control. Evolution at least to my mind attests to the miracle of human ingenuity. It is a recognition of not how far we have come but how much further we have still to go.

Though "Sabita" was able to tolerate her mother's behavior, thanks in part to the attitudes she learned within her joint family, and though she may even have managed to partially understand that behavior, she remains incapable of forgiving her mother for a perceived lack of parenting skills. In this respect, it seems to me that "Sabita" is perhaps lacking in generosity of spirit. Has her mother truly done her a grave injustice? This is an issue that she will have to sort out for herself in the fullness of time.

Knowing "Sabita" for as long as I have, I would say that she is only just beginning to see a true reflection of herself in the mirror. I do not know how long she will continue to cycle in and out of periods of stability. Her prognosis remains guarded until she becomes a permanent fixture at AA meetings.

The Twelve Steps program of AA presents a set of extremely workable spiritual principles. They form the basic template for recovery in a number of settings and have helped untold millions around the globe. They may be able to help "Sabita" keep her substance abuse problem in check, but her overall stability will likely remain at issue for quite some time because her psychological dependency will not be easy to overcome. Precious few people understand themselves in anything other than abstract terms, and "Sabita" is no exception. Her attempts at coming to grips with who she is are modest at best.

The causes of BPD are still very much a subject of debate. In most cultures, the social identity of a man and his persona are less dependent on his attachment figures than they are for women. This may be one reason we see fewer true personality disorders among males. There are some notable exceptions however, to be discussed later.

With respect to the strained relationship "Sabita" had with her mother while growing up and whether it may have caused her Borderline Personality Disorder to develop, I will add that in many societies, women typically govern relationships, in part because of their innate physiology, in part by right of their motherhood role. As "Sabita's" mother forfeited this right due to the circumstances under which the marriage occurred and was propagated, "Sabita's" sense of what womanhood actually represents is perhaps arguably skewed.

Tying together the psychospiritual and the clinical elements brought together thus far, the central point I would like to make is that while one's fundamental identity is in fact a composite of several influences; paramount amongst these is an appreciation of spiritual clarity. In this regard, the creation myths discussed at the beginning of the chapter help place into context man's relationship with both himself and his immediate environment, but more so, his orientation to the cosmos. This latter relationship is pivotal, as is the fact that for people to understand it, they must first and foremost be anchored within themselves, for the doorway to other dimensions is an inner one. This is the great realization that the Upanishads had codified already in the 8th century BCE.

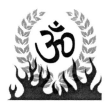

CHAPTER 6

HISTRIONIC PERSONALITY DISORDER

"There comes a time in every man's life,
and I've had plenty of them."

– Casey Stengel

"Lana" has a history of depression dating back many years and has sought medical attention for this condition with some success. In fact, she attempted suicide while she was under my care and was hospitalized. When questioned about it, she said that she had simply done something "stupid."

A vital piece of information concerning this attempt is that "Lana" and her husband were not getting along. He is an alcoholic, and I have a suspicion that too much alcohol likewise precipitated "Lana's" suicide attempt though she has never openly discussed her drinking habits with me. I gathered that she and her husband had separated and were both in counseling. I do not know all the reasons for the break-up or whether a reconciliation was in the works, but I do know there were young children involved.

"Lana" is someone who manifests prominent histrionic traits in addition to a possible underlying mood disorder and a substance abuse disorder. Histrionic Personality Disorder (HPD) is characterized by pervasive attention-seeking behavior including inappropriate sexual seductiveness and shallow or exaggerated emotions. The histrionic personality is highly expressive and emotional, so it is difficult to say at what point a true HPD manifests, but knowing "Lana" as well as I now do, I would say that she has definitively crossed the line. I suspect that someone she trusted abused her sexually at a young age.

The core issue "Lana" has struggled with in life has been her inability to give and receive love. She exhibits unduly rigid boundaries or personality walls. On a subconscious level, her deepest fear is perhaps the fear of intimacy due to the fact that she has not yet come to terms with the anger and rage she feels at having been victimized as a child. As we shall see, this suspicion was indeed borne out during the course of our sessions together.

"Lana's" first line of defense should be to come to terms with the chemical dependency she may be harboring so that she can then begin addressing any underlying mood disorder that may coexist. It is impossible to make a diagnosis of mood disorder when it is overlaid by an untreated chemical dependency.

To be more specific, "Lana" needs to "dry out" and open the door to a conscious reflection of her true emotions and their underlying significance. Therapy remains an option for her, but she should seek the services of a female psychotherapist to discuss her issues as there are bound to be transference difficulties with a male therapist. "Transference" is the projection of subconscious material on to a therapist of the opposite sex, which "Lana" would be likely to do owing to her past experiences of sexual abuse.

Where a concurrent substance use disorder exists, medication is sometimes an option, as is an abstinence-based recovery program, often coupled with self-help groups. However, when an individual has been properly medicated and his or her addictive behavior appropriately addressed, psychotherapy remains the only accepted option to treat the underlying personality issues involved. As mentioned, "Lana's" core issue is a difficulty in giving and receiving love. Perhaps this is the subconscious justification for the pervasive attention-seeking behavior she manifests.

There is a continuum of human behavior such that, depending on the context in which an individual's behaviors are manifest, they may be classified as either normal or pathological. What led me to the conclusion that "Lana" was indeed histrionic was the fact that both her suicide attempt and the context in which it occurred suggested additional psychiatric disorders that had not yet been addressed. For one thing, on numerous occasions in my office, she would burst into a tantrum for no apparent reason. These shallow outbursts clearly indicated that she herself was perpetuating the misery in her life, but no amount of rationalization on my part to eliminate her self-limiting beliefs and false ideas seemed to help.

In all honesty, I must say that I gave up trying after a while and "Lana" ultimately went looking for sympathy elsewhere, much to my delight. However, to my surprise, she returned within a few months, requesting that I again see her as a patient. I realized later that my practice of maintaining firm boundaries – neither overly rigid nor flimsy – helped her to contain her emotions and express herself in a therapeutically beneficial manner. This transpired even though the subject of her sexual abuse was never broached in these sessions.

As it turns out, "Lana" and her husband ultimately separated, which was perhaps a good thing as the marriage had remained loveless. In the months that followed, "Lana" experienced extreme difficulty in connecting at an emotional level with someone of the opposite sex, though outwardly she appeared to be an intelligent, attractive and cheery individual. She could not understand why.

Much later, we began to explore "Lana's" deeper issues. The insight-oriented psychotherapy and cognitive behavioral therapies that had been recommended for her had remained entirely unproductive. Somewhat exasperated and at a loss for a definitive course of action, I encouraged her to take up yoga.

Over the sessions that followed, as "Lana" began to take a keen interest in yoga, she reported episodes where she would experience spontaneous outbursts of emotion for no apparent reason. In therapy, she had always associated these flare-ups with whatever she happened to be discussing at the time, which was by and large totally innocuous. In the context of her involvement with yoga, however, "Lana" came to understand that her outbursts were indeed not only unjustifiable but unsubstantiated.

Almost a year after starting yoga, "Lana" informed me that she had grown up in an incestuous family and had been molested repeatedly by her older brother. After confiding in me, she broke down and I sensed that a deep burden had been lifted from her soul. At the same time, I realized that the environment in which she had been raised, where unduly rigid boundaries had been the rule, had preempted "Lana" from coming to terms with her emotional pain.

In the older societies of the East, there is an entrenched notion that health is best defined in positive rather than negative terms. This perhaps reflects the fact that Eastern medicine is based on controlled observation over a prolonged period of time rather than on dissection and experimentation as it has been in the West. Eastern medical concepts are also arguably more holistic. They incorporate the notion of an innate intelligence that is recruited during the healing process rather than simply relying on drugs that by and large interfere with the body's natural mechanisms.

When I was an undergraduate student at university, I took a course entitled History of Medicine. One of the treatises I read during that course was Sir William Harvey's *Anatomical Treatise upon the Movement of the Heart and Blood in Animals*, written in 1628. To reiterate, much of Western medical understanding of disease today is rooted in centuries-old observations and the laws of motion postulated by Sir Isaac Newton over three hundred years ago. For example, our understanding of and the management of illnesses like ischemic heart disease remain predominantly mechanical to this day. The same holds true as concerns mental illness. Freud's concept of libido or lust is based on Newton's idea of "blind" universal energy.

The longer I practice medicine, the more I become aware that every treatment modality comes with implicit assumptions. In his best-selling book, *Ageless Body, Timeless Mind*, author Dr. Deepak Chopra lists and subsequently refutes ten assumptions upon which the traditional model of mainstream medical care is based.

Needless to say, there have been many advances in the field of medicine. One particularly promising one is that the mind is now considered an invisible if not ubiquitous field, comprising as such the invisible software that creates and controls the functioning of the physical body. One exciting application of this new understanding is the introduction and use of meditative techniques to treat a number of chronic illnesses including both mental illnesses and addictions. In North America, the shift began about a century ago with the grassroots movement that would later blossom into the first self-help fellowships. Today, a number of well-known specialized health centers are officially using mind-body awareness techniques like Transcendental Meditation to treat a diverse range of chronic ailments.

As for solving the problem of dual diagnosis, I contend that early recognition and intervention are key as the condition is entirely treatable. There is a growing body of evidence both in favor of and against traditional allopathic treatments, and in an effort to forestall adverse public opinion, mainstream medicine is becoming increasingly evidence-based. At the same time, funding for the extensive clinical trials required to bring new medications to market is more and more being provided by the multinational pharmaceutical conglomerates. More applications are surely in the offing despite the cost hurdle.

Still, it often occurs to me as I go about my daily practice that the entire knowledge contained in the *Diagnostic and Statistical Manual of Mental Disorder-IV* represents but a fraction of man's collective knowledge. We perceive mental illness along a continuum, and the tide of prevailing medical knowledge turns every 10 to 15 years. Old concepts are replaced by new ones and evidence in support of the paradigm shift springs up to accompany it in a timely fashion. So it would seem that mental illness does not exist as an absolute but only in relative terms. Let's take a look at a case to that effect.

"Howard" is 54 years of age. He was diagnosed with Bipolar Disorder, Type 1 in 1992. He was placed on antipsychotic medication and his psychosis resolved. He was given a dual diagnosis shortly thereafter and placed in an abstinence-based monitored recovery program. He graduated from this to self-help recovery after five years.

After twelve years in recovery, "Howard" started having a shot of alcohol now and then as the occasion arose. I informed him that his recovery was abstinence-based at this point and explained to him the nuances of the term.

He understood and acknowledged the importance of self-control. He remains stable in this regard with respect to his chemical dependency. By this I mean that he does have the occasional drink but remains vigilant. In "Howard's" case, it would seem the higher cortical centers of the brain have over-ridden the lower centers within the brainstem where subliminal impulses are generated and acted upon. This phenomenon, termed self-regulation, is still not entirely understood and remains an area of active study.

After many years of stability, "Howard" informed me that he wished to taper his dose of antipsychotic medication. When I asked why, he stated that he simply wondered whether he still needed to take it. I advised against this measure, carefully explaining to "Howard" that the prevailing body of medical evidence weighs heavily in favor of lifetime treatment with antipsychotic medication for individuals with Bipolar Disorder, Type 1. This is especially true of those who have a documented history of psychosis, which "Howard" did.

A year later, "Howard" informed me that he had tapered and ultimately discontinued his medication against medical advice. He had remained stable during this interval with regular follow-up. He asked me why he had not suffered a recurrence of psychotic symptoms. My response was to turn the question around and ask him how he thought he had managed to accomplish this feat. He simply said, "Faith!"

Just so it is clear, the issue here is neither mental illness nor addiction but spiritual clarity. How *does* one overcome dependency? Clearly, "Howard" had come to terms with this issue. Overcoming his dependency through growth on the spiritual plane, "Howard" had understood intuitively who he was, and this understanding crystallized despite any of the labels and concepts currently used to qualify him. It has taken almost twenty years of treatment and several hospitalizations for him to arrive at this understanding of himself. Is it a valid representation? Well, given the fact that he no longer requires medication, continued observation is all that is warranted and time will tell.

The point I am making with "Howard's" case is that it would seem that "mind over matter," if not "faith over matter," does have its place in recovery. Ideally, strong personal values and beliefs should be instilled from an early age in the home, which can then be reinforced through education. One's culture plays a pivotal role in this regard. For many, religion does as well. One's experiences in life also have a bearing on the inherent wealth or poverty of one's spiritual beliefs and one's ability and openness to experience "faith" as a dimension of recovery. Dr. Gabor Maté includes an excellent discussion of such issues in his book, *In the Realm of Hungry Ghosts*.

Unfortunately, the tide of medical research weighs heavily in favor of the pharmaceutical giants. Drugs do seem to count for a lot. However, there is scarcely 20 or 30 years of cumulative experience with some of the newer pharmaceutical agents used in the treatment of most psychiatric conditions. Certainly, there is often an improvement in the quality of life for patients treated with these agents, but what are the real end points being measured? Under what circumstances do mechanisms of natural healing take precedence? In my opinion, this question has not yet been studied in any convincing detail despite its being a core issue.

We have now met "Lana" and "Howard," and have had a glimpse of some of the difficulties involved in trying to establish spiritual clarity in a therapeutic relationship. Let me now add some fuel to the fire by raising more dual diagnosis issues that need exploring.

"Rachel" walked into my downtown clinic seeking the services of a doctor willing to take on transgendered patients. Not being experienced in this particular field of medicine, I reluctantly agreed to her request simply because I sensed her pain and empathized. When we first met, she had not yet begun the process of transitioning between sexes. In medical terms, "Rachel" suffered from Gender Identity Disorder, believing she was a female in a man's body. This disorder occurs within the context of a much larger issue which is termed Gender-related Dysphoria. Clearly, "Rachel" had deep-seated issues.

Gender Identity Disorder (GID) is extremely rare, with a worldwide lifetime prevalence of about 0.001% to 0.002%. The reason I see this disorder more frequently than most general practitioners is that I work in a clinic in a large metropolitan area that harbors and supports alternate lifestyles. Nonetheless, specializing as I do in the treatment of addictions and mental health issues, my role as regards GID remains basically supportive.

It took me approximately a dozen encounters with "Rachel" to understand who she was. During this time, she successfully transitioned between the sexes. However, at the end of it all, I did not feel that I had actually accomplished much. I say this simply because she told me the following rather candidly:

I do not feel that God helped me through my transition at all. I think that if I hadn't come from a religion that told me I would burn in hell for what I was doing, I probably would have come out at a very early age. Either God doesn't care about us and we are free to be who we naturally are, or God does care one heck of a lot and freedom is something we must first comprehend and then go about the business of earning.

My take on what "Rachel" expressed was basically that she had yet to come to terms with her pain. In many ways, she had done so intellectually, physically and perhaps emotionally by completing her transition. Spiritually, however, she was a mess. Much of "Rachel's" life experience as a man prior to undergoing her transition had had to do with letting go of ideas, attitudes, beliefs and values that did not express who she knew herself to be in reality. The question of sexual identity added an extra layer of complication.

After a few visits, "Rachel" casually informed me that she had been preoccupied with and even contemplated suicide before her transition. However, the thought of dying as a man and being put on exhibition for all eternity in this way revolted her. She decided instead that she would spend every last dime on surgeries and hormones to try and get to a place where she could be free. If she remained unhappy having reached this place, she would then commit suicide.

Prior to sexual reassignment surgery (SRS), "Rachel" was required to undergo a readiness assessment conducted by a registered psychologist. Having glanced at the assessment, which was supportive of her transition, I realized that the accepted standard of care for her was in fact substandard. To me, "Rachel" not only manifested Gender Identity Disorder, which is perhaps qualified given how despondent she was over her assigned sex, but even more deeply-seated was an underlying Histrionic Personality Disorder that remained to be addressed. The issue was, should it have been addressed before the sexual reassignment surgery?

I am fully aware that one cannot make the same categorical statements about HPD within the transgendered context as one typically might when it is clustered with other Cluster B personality disorders. So that all individuals ultimately receive the most appropriate psychotherapeutic services, it would take a new framework by which to gauge a patient's situation and understand the underlying psychodynamics involved.

According to Upanishadic thought, already in the 8th century BCE, all the gods, all the goddesses and all the worlds are within us. When viewed from this vantage point, the mind becomes a stage where the forces of conflict are played out in dramatic fashion to a foregone conclusion.

A perfect illustration of this transformation occurs in Hindu mythology, where the mother goddess Durga, the personification of the life force, has the capacity to transform into many other goddess-figures while still maintaining her identity. One of them is the benign mother goddess Parvati. Another is the wrathful, almost demonic Kali, who represents the ultimate alienation of the self from its true self.

In the transformation myth, there is a scene where Kali does battle with an army of demons and loses her mind from the bloodlust. It is her consort Shiva who restores Kali to sanity, thereby transforming the mother goddess energy back to its benign form as Parvati. The story ends with Lord Shiva's immortal dance that occurs at both the beginning and the end of manifest creation. To me, he represents the central point within consciousness where all apparent motion stops and the gift of inner vision or spiritual clarity manifests.

I see in "Rachel's" story a modern retelling of the myth. I have spoken with her on occasion since her sexual reassignment surgery, and it is evident to me that she may know *what* she is, but she still hasn't figured out *who* she is. I do not wish to imply that all transgendered individuals are histrionic. However, as the transformation myth suggests, many GIDs do experience conflict that manifests as confusion, the remedy for which is to achieve spiritual clarity.

It seems to me that one's identity – which is a reflection of the degree of spiritual clarity that one has achieved – should be considered independent of gender. I do not believe that underlying conflict can be truly resolved until one has come to terms with the emotional pain that one is experiencing in life. I suppose that transitioning to another sex represents a degree of self-realization, but to my mind, it does little to resolve the underlying problem.

Why not? Well, I for one believe that being given a new body does not change all that much in the long run, at least in "Rachel's" case. I do not see her with any regularity now that she has successfully transitioned, but I would hazard a guess that she will experience some further mental health issue related to the pain unresolved at the core of her dysfunctional personality.

And what is the source of this pain? Gender seems to be the issue, but if the transformation myth is any indication, the real problem stems from the fact that it is "Rachel's" identity that remains ambiguous more than her sex-gender. In all likelihood, she will have tremendous difficulty making it through the final stages of the transitioning process.

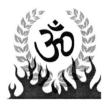

CHAPTER 7

ANTISOCIAL PERSONALITY DISORDER

"God writes a lot of comedy... the trouble is, he's stuck with so many bad actors who don't know how to play funny."

– Garrison Keillor

So far in this book, I have emphasized the importance of self-knowledge and faith in coming to terms with a dual diagnosis, and how to facilitate spiritual clarity in a clinical context to help deal with it. "Spiritual clarity" is not just a label: inasmuch as it helps to consolidate a positive understanding of self in the client, it assists the clinician most powerfully in his or her therapeutic initiative.

Faith does not easily lend itself to discussion on purely intellectual grounds. Nor do I attach any religious connotation to the word. As mentioned in an earlier chapter, faith serves as a bridge between intuition and self-knowledge insofar as the mind is transcended and awareness manifests. This process reflects a certain amount of integration within an individual's personality, the goal being a state of wholeness. Ultimately, faith embraces one's sense of spirituality in whatever way, shape or form that spirituality manifests.

Similarly, spiritual love or *agape* is an ideal. Yet, I consider it to be a true panacea in the fields of addictions and mental health. How so? Because the degree to which spiritual love is manifest within an individual's life often represents the extent to which psychological dysfunction has been transcended and wholeness achieved.

Another aspect of integration is *gnani* or "knowing." Gnani yoga is a discipline by which the practitioner pursues knowledge primarily to facilitate the growth of awareness. I have begun where appropriate to share some of its principles and wisdom in my clinical practice, and met with astonishing results. It tends to deepen the faith of an individual as he or she engages in the therapeutic process.

Awakening represents the finest flowering of a lifetime. The individual comes to terms with what has thus far been just a shadow of reality in the concrete world and grasps the presence of an inner reality. In turn, this new-found self-realization breeds an attitude of courage in the face of adversity, which is why it has been said that faith is the opposite of fear. As a clinician experienced in psychospiritual medicine, I can definitely attest to seeing this transformation in my patients.

Let me tell you about "Victor," a young man I have treated on and off for several years who approached me initially to get on my methadone program. During his first visit to the clinic, he told me he was purchasing 60 mg of street methadone daily but continued to inject "speedballs," a mixture of heroin and cocaine, with some regularity. When asked if he thought it prudent to increase his dose of methadone, he declined, stating that he was functioning well for now on the current dose and managing to hold down a steady job. As it turns out, this was quite an accomplishment for him.

I agreed to grant "Victor" entry into my methadone program in the interest of Harm Reduction, but after a few months a problem surfaced. His urine was testing sporadically positive for opiates other than methadone metabolites and it was turning up consistently positive for cocaine. This continued for a couple of months more, so I confronted "Victor" on the issue. He began to waffle and I gave him three months to clean up his act. At the end of the probationary period nothing had changed, so I wrote him a tapering script and discharged him from my program.

I suspected that "Victor" was basically addicted to crack and that he would shoot up when the opportunity arose. As his history bore out, he had little regard for the law or for the rights of others, which is a classic indication of Antisocial Personality Disorder (APD). So in "Victor's" case, the diagnosis seemed to perfectly fit the bill. Unfortunately, there is no recognized treatment for this disorder.

People with APD typically have no interest in learning from their mistakes, nor are they particularly concerned about their future. Totally consumed with immediate gratification, they are similarly uninterested in forming attachments to anyone or anything else. Most end up incarcerated or victims of addiction. Still, as an experienced clinician, I have come to realize that these statements about the disorder reflect only a half-truth. I have seen cases worse than "Victor's" turn over a new leaf.

Take "Marty," who is thirty years sober. He has had his fair share of hardship. He had one unsuccessful marriage when he was in the problem, and several others in sobriety. He has several children, all by different mothers, some of whom have not even acknowledged him as their father. He has been incarcerated numerous times but he feels vindicated as he received an official pardon.

"Marty" has the gift of the gab and can think on his feet. He is now a pensioner relying on the generosity of others for his daily bread, and he has got his act down to a fine art. Although he is the one getting monetary support, it is his benefactors who feel they are being helped.

"Marty" has devoted his entire life to the "selfless" support of the fellowship of AA since sobering up. Thirty years of attending meetings more or less twice a day has given him some measure of clarity. Today, "Marty" is a man of faith. His curious brand of spirituality is no doubt egocentric but it nonetheless reflects the fact that he has come to believe there is a God.

Still, "Marty" is by no means a saint. Despite the redeeming qualities he has developed, he is still riddled with character defects. In his favor, with over thirty years of recovery under his belt, he has helped numerous alcoholics and drug addicts turn their lives around. On the dark side, "Marty" understands very well that in order to get ahead in life by being on the take, one must give a little, too.

"Marty's" secret, if I may call it that, is to find ways to support others whenever the opportunity arises in order to increase the odds of keeping his pockets lined. Under the guise of helping them with their addiction, "Marty" has taken to the cleaners several financially endowed individuals that he has met through the fellowship. I understand this very well about "Marty" and tolerate his behavior within reason as he is basically a harmless vagrant who lives day to day believing in Divine Providence.

To the uninitiated, "Victor" and "Marty" may seem worlds apart. "Marty's" IQ is arguably higher than "Vic's," and in mellowing over the years, he has transitioned within medical parlance from being "vehemently antisocial" to being somewhat more "narcissistically inclined." However, there is often a significant degree of overlap as concerns these two disorders. On that score, "Victor" could benefit from some coaching from "Marty" because of the two disorders, NPD is less lethal.

Within a few months of his dismissal, I received notification that "Victor" was in pre-trial and slated to be placed on methadone. After serving his jail time and being placed on probation, he came back to see me requesting readmission to my methadone maintenance program. I agreed on condition that this time he follow my orders to the letter.

With time and compassionate care, "Victor's" use of drugs was gradually tapered to its current level. The cycle of repeated incarceration was curtailed and he achieved a degree of stability for the first time in his life. However, "Victor's" pattern of sporadically using remained problematic. I put it down to his having no constructive outlet for his frustration, and I believed him to be a suitable candidate for residential treatment. Had "Victor" agreed, I would have implemented this strategy. However, he did not.

"Victor's" demon ultimately declared itself when he one day confided a dark secret to me. It involved frequenting a local striptease establishment where he would invariably get loaded, using alcohol as the gateway drug to a repetitive cycle of behavior that caused his undoing on more than one occasion. Careful observation and interrogation over a protracted period of time eventually revealed the whole story. Once loaded, "Victor" would compulsively act out a violent sexual fantasy that involved raping a prostitute whilst under the influence of a mood-altering drug. More often than not, that drug was cocaine.

It should be clarified that "Victor" was an illegitimate child. His father was both physically and emotionally abusive and his mother was an enabler. His ex-wife would not tolerate his inbred disrespect of women and the marriage crumbled, ending in divorce. "Victor's" misogynistic attitude toward women subsequently hardened and became entrenched. It also reflects a deep-seated insecurity that he has not measured up to the mark in his father's eyes.

Psychoanalytically, "Victor" typifies an unresolved Oedipal Complex. As Freud initially coined this term, it refers to the stage of neurotic attachment where the child competes with the father for the mother's attention. When this stage remains unresolved, jealousy and rage become well-established.

My reading of the psychodynamics involved in this case is not solely based on a formal analysis of the client. It also takes into account my intimate familiarity with tantric rituals, which represent yet another form of yoga. Tantra has helped consolidate my understanding of "Victor" and others who are equally dysfunctional. For purposes of this discussion, let me state that in attempting to rise above his or her animalistic self through direct confrontation of its base tendencies, the tantric practitioner ultimately achieves a degree of self-realization.

In order to entice "Victor" to walk a spiritual path, I first appealed to his youthful ego, encouraging him to act on his desire to have sex but to do so while sober. This invitation was initially framed as a challenge to his manhood and he acquiesced. After several months of casual dating and casual sex, "Victor" became desensitized thanks to the process I had engaged him in and he revealed to me that he had become capable of ejaculating during sexual intercourse more or less at will.

Having experienced passion without any proclivity towards blind lust, "Victor" then realized that previously, when he was under the influence of both alcohol and cocaine, intercourse aroused an orgiastic frenzy within him that could only be relieved through some expression of violence. He chose a sex trade worker as sexual partner and his subsequent refusal to pay for services rendered most often led to trouble.

Having achieved a degree of satisfaction about his virility, "Victor" was able to transition to the next stage and confront his demon at last. Can his realizations be construed as a measure of success? Well, "Victor" has been dating a young woman for some time now and the two are contemplating moving in together. His partner "Sandra" is fairly liberated sexually and enjoys acting upon his male-oriented fantasies involving domination, at least on the surface. Though the two occasionally smoke grass, they rarely engage in the social use of any hard drugs anymore. "Victor" does however remain on methadone maintenance therapy.

On the surface, it could appear that "Victor" has bent "Sandra" to his will and is using her, but the scenario also serves to fulfill her innate desire to submit to his charm. And so we have a match ostensibly made in heaven, at least in the boudoir. Given how "Vic" operates, I do not doubt that there is a tremendous degree of dysfunction at the heart of the relationship, but under the circumstances, I would venture to say that the arrangement is about as good as it gets.

"Victor" and "Marty" represent the extremes in a continuum of dysfunction. "Marty" has technically gone beyond the need for help. I believe he has realized that the only way he can help himself is to be of service to others. However, within the context of his dual diagnosis, I do not think "Marty" can ever be truly selfless: his sociopathic personality takes precedence over any true altruism.

"Victor" has been conditioned from a young age to hate himself, so it is perhaps no wonder that he has no regard for the law or for the rights of others. If he lives long enough, wisdom may ultimately prevail and he too will turn over a new leaf. Still, my clinical experience to date indicates that in the absence of medical attention, the odds of this occurring are fairly miniscule.

When I first started practicing Addiction Medicine, I would have lost sleep over many cases I now consider to be fairly routine. But having acquired a certain familiarity with both mental health and sexual health issues over the years, I am now content in knowing that I do my best in the clinic. In many cases, I am dealing with severe dysfunction that simply does not lend itself to resolution based on the traditional medical paradigm.

I have also come to realize that I am helping myself in my practice as well as my patients. Those who come to see me benefit if and when they can see themselves reflected with perfect clarity. It is up to me to set an example, and my own spiritual condition is of paramount importance in order for me to do so. In other words, the more I help myself, the more others benefit. It is only when I am spiritually fit that I can be of assistance to the individuals I see in my practice.

I would add, however, that while dysfunctional individuals can change, they usually do so only when they clearly see the need for change. Many end up clinging to their fears instead of moving forward. It is those who come to trust in themselves and have faith that can most take the needed steps to get better. This in turn helps me to better serve them. For some reason, and I do not know exactly why, there is a domino effect involved.

It is safe to say that dual diagnosis is something physicians must confront more and more these days in their dealings with patients. Many, however, are not spiritually equipped to deal with the reality of mental illness within the setting of addiction.

Harm Reduction is one prevalent strategy being espoused not only by individual practitioners but also as a public health measure in the broader community. It includes things like campaigning for legislation against drinking and driving, assuring the distribution of condoms in high schools, setting up vaccination campaigns against hepatitis B and creating safe sites for injection drug use.

Such initiatives are considered a plausible alternative to the societal ills that would likely propagate, not disappear, in the absence of such safeguards. The basic philosophy of Harm Reduction is that there is no right or wrong when it comes to the complex area of human behavior. It aims to mitigate rather than eradicate unlawful practices such as prostitution, drug trafficking and other criminal activities.

The intent of Harm Reduction is not to vilify the social conscience of mainstream society but to contain the damage attributable to so-called illicit activities. The economic burden they impose is reason enough.

The issue is what should be the acceptable standard of care? Are we to support an attitude of permissiveness within society on the one hand and still penalize those who fall between the cracks on the other? This to me seems unconscionable.

Ultimately, in order to be successful, rehabilitation must be a collaborative effort. On the one hand, legislators need both the justification and a clear mandate to enact policy changes. On the other, policy changes are needed to free up the economic resources necessary to change the social standards, which is particularly appropriate where these no longer reflect the norms of society.

For any of this to occur however, society must cast off its cloak of pride, fear, rationalized avarice and sanctified misunderstanding. Public awareness is the key. Unfortunately, materialism and rampant individualism have been the cause of much undoing in Western society. Dual diagnosis is but one of the ever-rising social and spiritual costs.

In dealing with the dually diagnosed on an individual basis, I would re-iterate in closing this chapter that boundaries are a key concept. There is an increasing body of clinical evidence to this effect. Early in this work, I presented enmeshment and other early childhood scenarios from my own practice to illustrate how fundamentally important boundaries are in both understanding and treating the condition. But as I have also hoped to point out, the best outcome for the dually diagnosed goes way beyond strengthening the subject's ego through traditional psychotherapeutic measures to instill proper boundary differentiation: it stretches all the way to the subject then transcending that very ego. Allow me to explain further.

The ego is a vestige of the instinct to survive that has been evolutionarily conditioned into mankind's psyche. Certainly, it remains a key function and fulfills a valuable role when critical thinking, one's basic sexuality and aggression are required. However, the ego's mandate is best served when there is intense competition and selection pressure. Transcendence is, by definition, not something inbred. It occurs much higher in Maslow's Hierarchy of Needs, but that does not make it any less an existential urge. On the contrary, I believe that transcendence is the ultimate step in the self-actualization model advanced by Maslow. Transcendence resolves into wholeness, its ultimate goal.

Do I believe severe psychological dysfunction can be completely overcome? Well, in truth, the answer is "only partially" because precious few dually-diagnosed individuals actually make it to the final stage of recovery – spiritual recovery. However, it seems to me that if and when spiritual clarity has been achieved, a whole new dimension opens up: the prison of form identity is transcended and an aperture is created whereby the entire universe can be seen to be exploring itself through the individual. Before this can happen one must have both feet firmly planted upon this Earth.

And why is this relevant? Because the term "faith" can be substituted once clarity has been achieved, at which point and if permitted to do so, the same creative intelligence that oversees the entire workings of the universe can be seen to be operating within individual existence as well.

Having made this clarification, I suppose it goes without saying that I for one believe we live in a compassionate universe. I do not know for sure that there is a loving and merciful God at the helm, but I do know that the universe is intelligent. As the "fully automatic" model posits, which we discussed in Chapter 5, all of the odds are in our favor. Man is much more than simply an accident waiting to happen.

That said, I am at pains to explain why our ego-driven personalities strive to maintain the illusion of separateness, but they do. In modern man, this has created an anguished search for self that is readily apparent to any enlightened observer. To state the obvious antidote, one simple key to success in life is balance. Nowhere else is this need more poignantly reflected than in the context of dual diagnosis. Addiction is plainly and simply maladaptive behavior. Left unchecked, it inevitably becomes associated with mental duress, often leading to the diagnosis of mental illness in some shape or form.

I am now of the opinion, having practiced medicine for close to a quarter century, that mental illness and addiction are acculturated phenomena, meaning that they have developed through contact with another culture. One example of cultural clash is colonialism, which has led to the decimation of many of the world's great aboriginal peoples.

We have now reached a new turn on the spire, where modern popular culture is undermining many of the conventions traditionally held sacred within Western society. I am referring to such institutions as marriage and the family. The more our traditional value systems erode, the more core stability is fracturing in society as a whole. Not surprisingly, this trend is reflected statistically in the concurrent rise of addiction and mental illness.

My approach, if I may call it that, is to seek out and realign the patient's center so that his or her life again becomes rooted in the consciousness from whence it arose. Once the person is centered, intelligence of a higher order can be seen to be directing his or her actions, whatever name is ascribed to it.

Most individuals who have some familiarity with Twelve Step self-help fellow-ships are aware of the serenity prayer: *God, grant me the serenity to accept the things I cannot change, the courage to change the things I can, and the wisdom to know the difference.* I too believe that there is such a place where recovery, healing, balance and wholesomeness all begin. My term for this starting point is "faith."

When the mind is left alone and allowed to function in the way it was originally intended to do, something quite curious happens. Spaciousness is created. The controlling center that had sought to project itself into every conceivable situa-tion is dissolved once and for all, and henceforth, through a disciplined aware-ness, freedom manifests of a variety never before experienced. The inevitable end result is self-control.

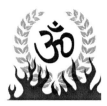

CHAPTER 8

SOME PERSONAL REFLECTIONS

*"Better keep yourself clean and bright; you are the window
through which you must see the world."*

– George Bernard Shaw

I hail from Goa, the smallest state in India. Located on the west coast, just to the south of Mumbai, it began as a collection of tiny fishing villages, but in the year 1498, the Portuguese arrived, and as they settled in, their language and customs permeated the local culture and deeply influenced its customs. They left fairly recently, in 1961, when Goa itself became an independent state within the Republic of India. Hindu, Christian and Moslem communities co-exist there peacefully now, creating a local subculture which is rather unique to the Indian subcontinent.

My wife Lucia Maria and I visit once or twice a year to vacation. She is still well-connected in Goa and we both enjoy dabbling in the local cuisine and social events. A unique mix of local seafood and old-world European charm, Goan cuisine boasts such exotic dishes as balchão, bacalhau, chorizo pão and vinda-loo, all of which tantalize even the most discriminating palate. My birthplace is also known for its fine beaches. I am proud to recommend it as a tropical paradise worth visiting!

Though of Goan heritage, I did not come to an awareness of the importance of my native culture until early mid-life. My parents both grew up under the British Raj, before India was divided by Partition. My father became a British citizen and worked in Hong Kong. This is where the family settled for the early part of my childhood. Old-world values prevailed such as honoring the Divine and the family first, but apart from that, our ways were rather Western. My mother tongue is English. I received the bulk of my primary education in an English public school, but I also have fond memories of India as I spent long periods of my childhood there living with my grandmother.

By contrast, my wife Lucia Maria was born and bred in Goa and her parents were both very traditional. The day began with morning mass and ended with the family saying the rosary around a statue of the Madonna. My father-in-law was educated in Portugal where he did his medical training and he later worked in Portuguese-occupied Angola as a military physician. My mother-in-law was both an exquisite hostess and an avid socialite as is the case in many well-to-do Goan households. At home, my wife spoke Konkani, an admixture of a local dialect of Sanskrit, Portuguese, Hindi and English, all of which are languages commonly spoken on the Konkan peninsula.

Although Lucia Maria and I were introduced in the formal, arranged manner whereby many Indian parents still chose spouses for their offspring, our decision to marry was very much our own. Still, when I first met her, I realized almost immediately that we would wed. I was a young man in many ways, but I knew already that her ability to adapt and acculturate would one day be an asset.

From spending so much time abroad, I myself knew little of Goan culture then, even though I was raised in a traditional Goan household. However, I did know that I was more Goan than non-Goan, and that was enough for me to decide to wed in accordance with the traditions of my native culture. Prior to seriously contemplating marriage, even before I met my future bride, I had already decided that what I most wanted in matrimony was the opportunity to grow in love. Having previously fallen in love Western-style as a bachelor, I knew the experience to be highly over-rated.

Almost three months to the date after our marriage, Lucia Maria was granted an entry visa to Canada and she became a permanent resident. Overall, the marriage was solid but it lacked passion. There were many reasons for this, but fortunately, all were remediable. We were both patient and slowly but surely, we warmed to one another and gradually became quite attached. At first, this made me feel rather uneasy, though I could not tell why. It then occurred to me that it was my wife's intention that I somehow change and become the person she had always dreamt of marrying.

In moving to Canada, Lucia Maria had gambled on love. Being younger than me and inexperienced in matters of the heart, she had thrown herself upon the sacrificial pyre, to use a colloquial Hindu expression. True, she had married within caste, but she did so against her parent's better judgment, making a leap of faith that her choice would work out for the best. Once committed, she did her best to render my heart captive. What she had yet to understand was that I was first and foremost inwardly free.

My awakening had occurred some years prior to marriage when I attended a local weekend Vipassana retreat, which involves long periods of meditation and unfolds in complete silence. After the first session, I fled the ashram hall in terror, but halfway to the parking lot, I stopped, realizing that I had to return. I did, and with great difficulty, managed to make it through the weekend. By the time I emerged, however, I had discovered a new path within.

For the next few years, I practiced meditation rigorously and assiduously for at least an hour a day. Within three years, I self-realized. Were I to sum up the experience, I would say that I gained a new sense of spaciousness in my being that created room for more growth to occur. Within any spiritual discipline, it is essential to experience a sense of one's own depth since impermanence, like waves on water, is a basic fact of life. And if all life is fundamentally sorrowful, the serenity provided by this deep knowing gives one an anchor and tempers the inevitable ebb and flow.

I then took up yoga, beginning with hatha yoga, the one most commonly known in the West. It teaches *asanas* or body postures to calm the mind, enhance concentration and build physical stamina. I then branched out into other, less physical and more reflective forms. Ultimately, I ending up being most drawn to gnani yoga, the yoga of knowledge, which teaches that absolute truth can be known through study and contemplation. Its basic tenet is "Know thyself." I discovered that to examine one's own thoughts and motivations and release the mind of preconceived notions creates an opening to behold the truth resting quietly within and find enlightenment.

Which is not, however, to forget my Christian spiritual roots. If you had asked me then what being a Christian means, I would have replied "to live by the example set by Christ." But I am no longer certain what many people today would make of this statement. So many are blinded by materialism and consistently make lifestyle choices that override if not shut down their Christ Center. Perhaps they are not even in touch with it.

My own journey home to the Father began when I realized that He alone was my best friend. Though I had everything as a young man, my cup always seemed half-empty. This led me down the path of self-destruction until one day I awoke, realizing at that exact moment and for the first time in my life how truly alone I was and how little faith I had. Like the Prodigal Son, I had come half-circle. Materialism had been my undoing too, but thanks to a loving and merciful God, I mended my ways and went about the business of living with renewed purpose.

My decision to return home to my native culture and marry within both caste and creed was an outward sign that I had acquired some wisdom in life and was ready to settle down, leaving behind my foolhardy and headstrong days as a young man. I had emerged knowing who I was, and I was beginning to realize that what I had always sought in marriage was companionship. I believed that above all else, the union of a man and a woman should be a blessed sacrament. Once I renounced my lesser ways, God saw fit to bless me with marriage, and sanctified the love that Lucia Maria and I shared.

After marriage, my professional responsibilities took on increasing significance. My health became my first priority, in the most inclusive sense of the word, and I attended to it dutifully. Soon, my spiritual health encompassed all other spheres, and as I became increasingly fit spiritually, my capacity to carry my fair share of the load also increased. I began to prosper.

I also began to understand wealth not materially but metaphorically. The greatest treasure I possessed was a profound and deep-seated sense of well-being, one that transcended who I was, granted me greater spiritual clarity and led me ultimately to a realization of wholeness. Wholeness is not a concept but a reality. By that I mean that it must be lived day-to-day rather than simply comprehended in abstract terms.

A further result of my having practiced meditation and yoga for many years is that I have become able to silence my mind. I no longer meditate but contemplate. The Japanese sage Koji Tse wrote in 1624: *A mirror not cluttered by dust shines brightly. The mind should be like that. Water not disturbed by waves settles down of its own. When what beclouds passes, happiness comes of its own.*

Meditation and yoga are tools used to silence the mind and hone the senses. Unfortunately, many people encounter mainly resistance, at least initially, when they try to do it. This stage passes, however, if one perseveres, and once silenced the mind can be applied at its maximal potential to whatever situations one encounters in life.

Aside from meditation and prayer, is there some objective, scientific way to bridge the gap between the inner and outer worlds? University of London physicist David Bohm, a protégé of Einstein and one of the world's most respected quantum physicists, proposed that objective reality does not exist, or rather that it is an illusion, somewhat like a hologram, subtended by a deeper level of reality. [1]

To understand Bohm's startling assertion, one must first understand a little about holograms, which are three-dimensional photographs made with the aid of a laser. To make a hologram, the object to be photographed is first bathed in the light of a laser beam. Then a second laser beam is bounced off the reflected light of the first, and the resulting interference pattern, the area where the two laser beams commingle, is captured on film. When the film is developed, it looks like a meaningless swirl of light and dark lines. But as soon as the developed film is illuminated by another laser beam, a three-dimensional image of the original object appears.

To enable people to better grasp the implications of holography, Bohm offers the following illustration. Imagine an aquarium containing a fish. Imagine also that you are unable to see the aquarium directly and that your knowledge about it and what it contains comes from two television cameras, one directed at the front of the aquarium, and the other at its side. As you stare at the two television monitors, you might assume that the fish on each of the screens are separate entities. After all, because the cameras are set at different angles, the images are different.

But as you continue to watch the two fish, you will eventually become aware that there is a certain relationship between them. When one turns, the other also makes a slightly different but corresponding turn. When one faces front, the other always faces toward the side. If you remain unaware of the full scope of the situation, you might even conclude that there must be two fish instantaneously communicating with one another, but this is clearly not the case.

According to Bohm, there is a connection between subatomic particles that is not only faster than light, but the harbinger of a deeper level of reality that we are not privy to, a more complex dimension beyond our own that is analogous to the aquarium. At that deeper level of reality, all things in the universe are infinitely interconnected, even time and space. Nothing is truly separate from anything else. And, he adds, we view objects like subatomic particles as separate from one another because we are seeing only a portion of reality. Like our TV monitor images of the fish, such particles are not separate "parts" but facets of a deeper, underlying unity that is ultimately as holographic and indivisible as we are.

And how does all of this apply in the case of dual diagnosis? Well, put simply, I believe we need to transcend any superficial understanding we may have of what is actually occurring at a neurobiological level and surrender, when it is appropriate, to the evidence. The mind is like a mirror. As it is gently polished, its fundamental clarity and brightness emerge. When dual diagnosis is resolved, some form of inner transformation has occurred, resulting in a tenable stability that neither waxes nor wanes over time.

Let us recall the words of our Japanese sage – that water not disturbed by waves settles down on its own and its true depth is fully appreciated. In physics, time and three-dimensional space should be considered part of a deeper and all-pervasive natural order that is self-regulating. As concerns amelioration and healing, once depth and clarity have been attained, stability should ensue as par for the course. I have thus far several clinical cases illustrating the nuances of dual diagnosis to support this contention.

What then is the role of medication? Administered by the inexperienced, most psychotropic medications suppress the individual's thinking and accomplish little more than a non-surgical lobotomy. The only advantage they offer is that they confine any disturbance to a particular level of consciousness, creating an acceptable standard of medical practice for society at large and a benchmark by which to empirically measure the claims of the pharmaceutical companies. Ethics dictate first and foremost that those individuals who have a mental illness be afforded treatment, and that those who are entrusted with providing it be competent in performing their duties. That said, ethics also dictate that patient health not be cast under the wheel of the market economy.

Sadly, as the concept is currently embraced within society, "health" has more or less become a commodity. The trend toward generic pharmaceuticals reflects this fact. However, while market forces and the manufacturing process have made medicines an easily accessible reality in many parts of the world, the conceptual advances that paved the way for these developments have long been overshadowed by the marketing aspect. It is a sad fact that many people in my generation prefer to "pop a pill" for a heart condition, for example, rather than addressing the smoking, lack of exercise and improper diet that caused the problem in the first place.

I would actually take that observation a step further and point out that much "dis-ease" begins in the mind. An estimated 85% of chronic ailments are the result of an aberration in one's patterns of thought, behavior and nutrition. [2] What this suggests is that balance is the order of the day. Yes, the practice of medicine has evolved into an art form, but more than just the skillful prescribing of medication, it should now be much more about educating the public.

For example, the discovery that omega-3-fatty acids are an effective mood stabilizer in the treatment of Bipolar Disorder was, for me, a landmark clinical trial. When viewed in conjunction with the underlying neurobiology of the disease [3], this development marks a breakthrough in understanding the condition at the biochemical level. Moreover and of equal or greater importance, it marks a paradigm shift in the currently-accepted standard of reputable medical practice, at least in my area of clinical practice, where there is an increasing incidence of iatrogenic illness (complication related to diagnosis and treatment of disease, regardless of whether the condition occurs as a known risk of a procedure or through errors of omission or commission). The older generation of mood stabilizers, for example, notoriously disturb thyroid, kidney and liver function, and patients must be monitored regularly for these disturbing side effects.

To reiterate, health should be an intrinsic goal of our social system rather than a commodity to be supplied by the market based on supply and demand. Of course, the private sector does need to be involved, and the degree to which subsidization occurs should reflect the resources, time and effort involved in bringing product or service improvements to the marketplace. Ideally though, research and development should be the impetus that drives the market economy, not profit.

For this to happen in reality, a differential tax structure needs to be put into place, and the model by which health care is provided needs to be revamped. One thing we know, and with all due respect to the endless ideological rants that stating the obvious can foment, privatization of health care doesn't work. It needs to be government-subsidized. Such, to put it bluntly, is the nature of the beast. However, we also know from experience that nationalizing health care using a fee-for-service model results in patients being over-diagnosed, over-prescribed and over-treated in an effort to maximize revenue and profit.

A capitation-based model – where there is also a shift in emphasis toward preventative health care – is an alternative, and it is the preferred model of health care provision in some European countries. But as it turns out, these countries are attracting fewer and fewer young graduates to their medical schools. Also, in order for the capitation model to work, individual health care providers must be able to evaluate the cost-effectiveness of a particular intervention so as to not exceed the budget allocation in managing their allotment of patients.

The added accounting could easily lead to an even higher burden of the bureaucratic minutiae that is already sapping the time and core focus of the practitioners working under such a model of health care provision. Furthermore, I for one do not accept that doctors be forced to take over the role of large insurance companies or sectors of the government that are better equipped to coordinate and manage the necessary infrastructure and administrative aspects of health care provision and to sustain the financial insolvency that typically arises through mismanagement.

One grassroots approach that can help pave the way to a broader-based solution is evidence-based medicine. The reality of clinical practice today is such that independent peer review is essential in order to ensure that the mandate of self-regulation enacted by the medical profession itself is enforced. Furthermore, evidence-based medicine will determine the accepted standard of care where pharmaceuticals are concerned, particularly as the existing tide of medical knowledge overturns itself approximately once every 10 to 15 years. Admittedly, there is much work yet to be done.

In the area of my specialty, dual diagnosis, another solution I wholeheartedly endorse is the platform of Harm Reduction, a basic extension of the Hippocratic Oath, whose primary mandate it is to do no harm. I have discussed this philosophy elsewhere in this book. However, I would add here that I believe it is the duty of the experienced clinician operating within the Harm Reduction paradigm to nonetheless "disturb" the individual client insofar as to challenge him or her to maximal potential. Yes, the Hippocratic Oath still exists, but the burden of care must also lie with the patient. With experience, it is indeed possible to gain the respect and admiration of the client while assisting him or her to define and own deeper levels of health and wellness.

The Addiction Medicine paradigm is well established more or less worldwide, and consists of three main phases. During the initial stages of acute stabilization, medication is often necessary, and a battery of laboratory investigations is required to define the scope of the problem and establish a baseline. Mandatory tests include viral serology to check for hepatitis A, B and C and HIV as well as a metabolic profile. Depending on the results, clients can be directed to other medical specialties as needed.

Acute stabilization is to be gauged by regular attendance at appointments and compliance with medication. Sometimes, residential treatment is indicated. Once initial stabilization has been achieved – a process that can require a year or longer in many cases and still remain tenuous – intermediate objectives can be outlined. These include finding stable housing, reintegrating into the workforce and successfully navigating the complexities of human relationships. These intermediate objectives often require from three to five years to attain, depending on the severity of the condition(s) present.

The final stage of recovery is spiritual recovery, which encompasses a very personal awakening and is typically life-long. Each recovery is unique, such that established paradigms fail at this point and the generalizations that characterize them begin to break down. The innate intelligence of each individual is to be truly appreciated. At this stage, the Addiction Medicine paradigm is to be augmented. For this purpose I use the term Psychospiritual Medicine, which itself is an area of evolving specialty. For more information on this specialty, I suggest Dr. Deepak Chopra's work, *Ageless Body, Timeless Mind,* written almost two decades ago.

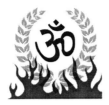

CHAPTER 9

A VISION FOR
CANADA'S DUALLY DIAGNOSED

"A hospital bed is a parked taxi with the meter running."

– Groucho Marx

In an excellent position paper, the National Coalition on Dual Diagnosis, formed in May 2008, released a policy statement which I think sums up quite succinctly many of the core ideas and opinions expressed to date in this publication. [1] Though the definition of Dual Diagnosis is somewhat different to that used here, one key point is the fundamental need for dually-diagnosed individuals to have equal access to medical services. The policy paper explains:

Many people with a dual diagnosis are misunderstood, cannot communicate, or are denied certain services. They may have access to some services, but outcomes will be poor unless services are designed to meet their particular needs.

The paper then goes on to enumerate factors present in the dually diagnosed that contribute to severe health inequity being exercised against them and, ultimately, to their marginalization. As both a primary care physician and a physician who specializes in the care of the dually diagnosed, I wholeheartedly concur that what this population needs is direct access to positive determinants of health such as adequate housing, nutrition, education, economic security, work, safe communities and social inclusion.

Realistically speaking, most if not all of these services are affordable to members of a disenfranchised population only if and when they are subsidized. Accordingly, within the current model, a primary health care provider must intervene on behalf of an individual with a dual diagnosis who has been marginalized, either through the progress of the addiction process or due to coexisting psychosocial and/or mental health issues. Such action is necessary in order to orchestrate and triage the individual through to the appropriate agencies so that these services can be accessed in a timely fashion.

My rather unique position and experience have afforded me the benefit of added insight that I will share briefly here, reiterating some of the statements made in the Coalition position paper by placing them into the context that is familiar to me while amending or expanding on others. For one thing, whereas the typical primary care physician would tend to address the problem of dual diagnosis by prescribing psychotropic medication, this measure, when viewed through the magnifying glass of specialized care, treats only the periphery of this condition, and thus represents only a band-aid solution to the growing problem of health inequity among Canada's dually-diagnosed subpopulation. Without an in-depth assessment of the underlying causes of the client's challenging behaviors, medication often does more harm than good, not just to the individual but in a widening circle of influence that includes his or her family and loved ones, health care providers and general social milieu with all the various levels of contacts that it entails.

Suppose for an instant that a dually diagnosed patient has obtained access to positive determinants of health. What then? Clearly, within a socialized system of health care, the human costs of the proffered services need to be weighed against the economic burden. And this is perhaps the crux of the matter. Just so the question is clear, a framework is required that evaluates the direct cost to Canadian society of institutionalized and tertiary care of the dually diagnosed versus the perceived "loss" of productivity return for this population as a whole.

Once a standard of established and reputable care is established, once the funds are "freed" and some portion allocated towards the creation of tailor-made services for the dually diagnosed, a community-based model of care can be put into place that highlights the role of prevention early on versus costly containment later. What kind of measures might that include? For one thing, an emphasis on early detection of issues affecting children and adolescents would lay the groundwork for an interdisciplinary approach to nipping the problem in the bud. For another, primary care physicians like GPs who work in walk-in clinics and family physicians could be cross-trained in basic treatment modalities for the dually diagnosed.

Treating the problem at the end of the road, when it has become entrenched, entails a host of very costly tertiary considerations such as long lead times for the training of specialists and the need for sophisticated facilities, equipment and other such infrastructure to name but a couple of ancillary issues. One of the most damaging consequences however is the long wait-time for patients to receive treatment. This one factor ultimately defeats the whole issue as many revert, while waiting, to the problematic behaviors that led them to seek assistance in the first place.

In sum, it seems to me that a community-based preventive care model would be more cost-effective in the long run than the one currently in place in some parts of the country. In British Columbia at least, the philosophy and practice of Harm Reduction are already well entrenched. Also, the College of Physicians and Surgeons of British Columbia has an established mandate to provide specialized training to licensed physicians so that the growing population of dually-diagnosed individuals can access the services which have been created to meet their specialized needs.

As far as implementation goes, what I think needs to be put into place at this stage is a three-tiered strategy. In line with the recommendations of the 2008 Coalition paper previously mentioned, the first tier would include an initial public awareness campaign informing Canadians that, in the Coalition's words:

People with a dual diagnosis are particularly vulnerable, stigmatized and marginalized. Nonetheless, they are citizens of this country, entitled to health equity and an equal opportunity to live and participate – with respect and dignity when and how they choose in Canada's communities.

As a second tier, an initiative coordinated at both the federal and provincial levels of government is essential, and it needs to target four general areas – health promotion and disease prevention at both the primary care as well as tertiary care levels. It may or may not be obvious, but allow me to belabor the point that most of the economic burden associated with dual diagnosis would be alleviated if the concept of health was defined positively and disease prevention rather than treatment were the key focus of this tier. From an economic perspective true savings would accrue if the quality of care were not compromised once the need for tertiary care is realized. At this stage we are talking about containment of the problem. Therefore, it is good management to allocate a significant portion of funds toward the amelioration of the problem at a primary care level. How?

Well, having worked in many sectors of health care over the years I would encourage policy makers to ensure that family practitioners be encouraged and supported by local self-governing bodies such as the jurisdictional medical colleges to meet an entirely different set of specific objectives aimed at curtailing rather than containing the problem of dual diagnosis and that medical practitioners who choose to work for convenience sake in walk-in-clinics recognize that in doing so they are servicing the needs of a population in transition during the initial implementation phases of this strategy. To this end I would encourage privatization of all walk-in-clinics and the imposition of regional levies for such clinics. The end result would be a shift at the level of primary care from the present standard of containment as witnessed by the currently escalating trend of underserviced elements of the general population. With such a shift at the level of primary care the entire notion of health promotion is being addressed.

The issue of disease prevention is to be addressed now in meeting the specific objectives alluded in the foregoing paragraphs. Once larger segments of the population are being serviced medically in a comprehensive fashion by encouraging these segments to seek out the services of qualified family practitioners trained to meet established targets by imposing a system-access fee for those who choose not to have a share in their health then in essence there will be a shift in priorities within the health care system.

Having addressed the topic of health promotion the next issue to address is disease prevention. This will accordingly affect the allocation of resources and funding of social programs aimed at achieving positive determinants of health; not just within a dual diagnosis framework but within a more comprehensive framework by which health care provision is administered.

Accordingly, I propose that the appropriate bodies – the federal regulatory commissions as well as the provincial and territorial ministries and the jurisdictional health authorities – allocate sufficient funds to allow for the creation of a Canadian Center for Policy Research on Dual Diagnosis, with provincial, territorial and regional arms. The center ideally should be nonpartisan and have as its primary mandate the collection of appropriate data which it would then distribute by means of a centralized electronic registry to its provincial, territorial and regional arms with the emphasis being on disease prevention.

The purpose of this data-sharing would be to allow for monitoring and evaluation of the various non-governmental agencies and governmental departments and initiatives created to implement the unilateral recommendations of the Center for Policy Research on Dual Diagnosis, in an effort to reduce the ancillary costs associated with providing health care to this subset of the Canadian population within the current containment-based model as opposed to a preventative framework being advocated.

It stands to reason that among the major stakeholder groups who would stand to benefit from such a program would be the various provincial, territorial and regional ministries currently governing health care provision that already receive federal transfer payments. A centralized registry could track comprehensive demographic health indices, not only nationally but also as a means to rapidly compare regional indices with established nationwide prevalence rates.

This in turn would permit a more accurate and transparent evaluation of policy initiatives at all levels of government. It would also be a means to elicit data on the true priority needs of this vulnerable minority group and enable the development and efficient delivery of community-based coordinated care initiatives with the emphasis being on both primary and secondary prevention at both primary and tertiary care levels.

What should the role of the private sector be in this endeavor? Well, ultimately the principal shareholder to whom the Canadian government is accountable is the Canadian people as a whole, irrespective of the level of governance, branch or policy-initiative involved. Therefore, I propose then an independent, multi-disciplinary, privately-appointed Commission be sanctioned as a moratorium to evaluate the merits of public ownership in such a program. The purpose of such a Commission is to ensure transparency within government and accountability to all segments of the Canadian population.

Collecting real-time data on regional trends and tracking the status of health equity measures for marginalized populations such as the dually diagnosed would ultimately not only attest to the perceived soundness of these governmental initiatives but would also provide input on the cost-effectiveness of the policy-initiatives involved. Having labored in the field for two decades, I for one believe that transparency should be the first order of the day.

At the end of the day no two medical practitioners are alike. Such a system inherently recognizes this fact but also acknowledges that different segments of the medical system should have different agendas and monetary reward should be a function of the quality and not the quantity of the work which is performed. This is perhaps a reflection of the fact that clear objectives are to be outlined and targeted in a staggered fashion within such a strategy. That is not to say that one cannot work as much as or as little as they desire. However, financial remuneration at all levels of this system is based upon merit and productivity, reflecting the models entrenched roots within a system of social democracy.

To this end, private companies should not only be allowed to compete with government agencies, they should be encouraged to provide the products and services necessary to manage the dually-diagnosed population as competitively as is possible. Take as an example the condition of hepatitis C. In Canada compliance with treatment runs at an estimated 85% whereas in the States the rate is closer to 50%. Why? Well, in Canada the pharmaceutical companies provide education and support for individuals under treatment for this condition by training and providing qualified nurse practitioners to individuals who are being treated for the condition. I also think that genericization of pharmaceuticals should be encouraged particularly as concerns the needs of Canada's geriatric population which currently consumes the most medication, where the evidence suggests such a practice is appropriate; and where it does not, as for example with many of the comorbid conditions associated with dual diagnosis like coinfection, licenced practitioners should be allowed the discretion to prescribe pharmaceuticals currently under patent with a relaxation of the regulatory standards currently in place restricting the use of these substances.

After all once the final phases of such a strategy have been implemented the focus will be upon prevention and containment will no longer be the center of such a strategy. As far as long term objectives of such a strategy are concerned, the main aim of this strategy is to allow Canada's population to grow old gracefully. This aim will be achieved when health care provision is administered comprehensively with specific objectives in mind concerning the appropriate indices of population health to all segments of Canada's population.

At the end of the day, there are three great advantages to this arrangement. Both the private and public sectors become accountable to the Canadian people in real time, transparency is assured, and real-time data compiled by the central registry both informs and drives the recommendations of the Center for Policy Research. In addition, best use is made of modern technological resources that were not available when many of the current treatment models were devised. In turn, the Center keeps a steady hand on the helm, and thus do well-founded policy initiatives get enacted at the various levels of government involved. Cost-effectiveness reigns. In sum, this is a strategically-coordinated plan for the optimization of health care provision to Canada's dually diagnosed.

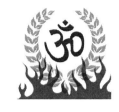

CONCLUSION

"All that is gold does not glitter, not all those who wander are lost.

The old that is strong does not wither, deep roots are not reached by the frost.

From the ashes a fire shall be woken, a light from the shadows shall spring.

Renewed shall be blade that was broken, the crownless again shall be king."

– J. R. R. Tolkien

The many faces of dual diagnosis …

Boundaries …

Awareness …

Faith …

Self-knowledge …

Values and belief systems …

Harm Reduction …

The Canadian health care system …

These are a few of the themes that have formed the tapestry of this book. My larger intent has been to show that spirituality does have a role to play, not only for the dually diagnosed client, but increasingly within the clinical sector itself and Addiction Medicine in particular. I have ended with the vision of a new model of care for dually-diagnosed patients. Essentially, what is involved is bringing medicine up to par with recent scientific discoveries and technological advances. I hope these reflections have served you well and I thank you for journeying with me.

Robert Pereira, MD

January 2011

CHAPTER 1

1. Kessler, Ronald C. "The epidemiology of dual diagnosis." Biological Psychiatry. 2004. Volume 56: issue 10: 730-737.

2. RachBeisel, Jill, Jack Scott and Lisa Dixon. "Co-occurring Severe Mental Illness and Substance Use Disorders: A Review of Recent Research." Psychiatric Services 50: (November 1999) 1427-1434.

3. Anecdotal evidence suggests that this relationship between "belief in a power greater than oneself" and "stability" has been accumulating since the advent of the first self-help fellowships almost a century ago. However, whether this relationship exists in the case of mental illness *per se* remains a point of some contention to this day.

4. Tacey, D. *Jung*. London. Granta Publications. 2006.

5. American Psychiatric Association. *The Diagnostic and Statistical Manual of Psychiatric Illness - IVR (DSM-IVR): Diagnosis, Etiology and Treatment*. Washington, DC: American Psychiatric Publishing, Inc., 2004.

6. Neighbors, Brian, Tracy Kempton and Rex Forehand. "Co-occurrence of substance abuse with conduct, anxiety, and depression disorders in juvenile delinquents." Addictive Behaviors. 1992. Volume 17: issue 4: 379-86.

7. Boden, J.M., D.M. Fergusson and L.J. Horwood. "Anxiety disorders and suicidal behaviours in adolescence and young adulthood: findings from a longitudinal study." Psychol Med. 2007; 37:431-440.

8. Turner, E.H., A.M. Matthews, E. Linardatos, R.A. Tell and R. Rosenthal. "Selective publication of antidepressant trials and its influence on apparent efficacy." N. Engl. J. Med. (January 2008) 358 (3): 252–60.

9. Maté, Gabor. *In the Realm of Hungry Ghosts: Close Encounters with Addiction*. Toronto: Vintage Canada, 2009.

10. Maté, Gabor. *Scattered Minds: A New Look at the Origins and Healing of Attention Deficit Disorder*. Toronto: Vintage Canada, 2000.

11. Robinson, David J. *The Personality Disorders Explained*. London, Ontario: Rapid Psychler Press, 2003.

12. Ibid.

13. Weisman, M.M., R.C. Bland, G.J. Canino et al. "The cross national epidemiology of obsessive compulsive disorder." Journal of Clinical Psychiatry, 1994: 55, 5-10.

14. Koran, Lorrin M. "Obsessive-Compulsive Disorder: An Update for the Clinician." Focus, 2007:(5):3.

15. *A Beautiful Mind*. Film directed by Ron Howard. Written by Akiva Goldsman. Image Entertainment. USA. 2001.

16. Kessler, Ronald C. "The epidemiology of dual diagnosis." Biological Psychiatry. 2004. Volume 56: Issue 10: 730-37.

17. National Coalition on Dual Diagnosis. *Dual Diagnosis Position Paper*. 2008. http://care-id.com/images/File/Position statement.pdf

CHAPTER 2

1. Martin, Paul. *Sex, Drugs & Chocolate: The Science of Pleasure*. London: Fourth Estate, 2008. ISBN 978-0-00-712708-5

2. Salyard, A. "On Not Knowing What You Know: Object-coercive Doubting and Freud's Announcement of the Seduction Theory." Psychoanalytic Review. 1994. 81(4): 659-676.

CHAPTER 3

1. Regier, D.A., M.E. Farmer et al. "Comorbidity of Mental Disorder with Alcohol and Other Drug Abuse. Results from the Epidemiologic Catchment Area (ECA) Study." JAMA 1990; 264: 2511-18.

2. Kessler, R.C., K.A. McGonagle and K.S. Zhao. "Lifetime and 12-month Prevalence of DSM III-R psychiatric disorders in the United States. Results from the National Comorbidity Survey." Arch Gen Psychiatry 1994; 51: 8-19.

3. Stohler, R., W. Rossler (eds). "Dual Diagnosis. The Evolving Conceptual Framework." Bibl Psychiatr. Basel, Karger, 2005. No. 172, pp. 105-14.

CHAPTER 5

1. Davy, Adams and A. Merry. *A Man Before Others: Rudolf Steiner Remembered*. Bristol: Rudolf Steiner Press, 1993.

2. A.H. Maslow. "A Theory of Human Motivation." Psychological Review 50(4) (1943):370-96.

CHAPTER 8

1. David Bohm. *Unfolding Meaning: A Weekend of Dialogue with David Bohm*. London: Routledge, 1996.

2. Chopra, Deepak. *Ageless Body, Timeless Mind: The Quantum Alternative to Growing Old*. New York: Three Rivers Press, 1994.

3. Manji, Husseini K et al. "The underlying neurobiology of bipolar disorder." World Psychiatry. 2003. October 2 (3): 136-146.

CHAPTER 9

1. National Coalition on Dual Diagnosis. *Dual Diagnosis Position Paper*. 2008. http://care-id.com/images/File/Position statement.pdf

The following resources are located for the most part in Vancouver and the Lower Mainland of BC. While current at the time of writing, the information is subject to change.

MENTAL HEALTH

Canadian Mental Health Association
1200-1111 Melville Street, Vancouver
604-688-3234

Mental Health Emergency Line
604-874-7307/527-0009

COUNSELING AND ADVOCACY

Advocacy Access Team
(counseling information and referral services)
BC Coalition of People with Disabilities
204-456 West Broadway, Vancouver
604-872-1278

Advocacy Group
1130 Jervis Street, Vancouver
604-683-4287

Battered Women's Support Services
(address withheld)
604-687-1868 (business/general line)
604-687-1867 (crisis line)

Community Volunteer Income Tax Program
(free income tax returns)
1-800-959-8281
www.cra.gc.ca/volunteer

First United Church
(advocacy, free income tax returns)
320 East Hastings Street, Vancouver
604-681-8365

Friends for Life
(support groups for life-threatening illnesses and grief counseling)
1459 Barclay Street, Vancouver
604-682-5992

ADULT DETOX SERVICES

Access Central: Easy Access to Detox
(Detox referral)
866-658-1221

Cordova Detox – Harbour Light
(referral through Access Central)
119 East Cordova Street, Vancouver
866-658-1221

Seniors' Well Aware Program
(community-based home detox program
for seniors)
212-309 West Cordova Street, Vancouver
604-662-7929
website: www.swapbc.ca
email: swap@123mail.org

Vancouver Detox
(referral through Access Central)
377 East 2nd Avenue, Vancouver
866-658-1221

ALCOHOL AND DRUG TREATMENT CENTERS

(programs are 4 to 6 weeks long)

Aurora Treatment Center (women)
5th Floor, 4500 Oak Street, Vancouver
604-875-2032

**Crossroads
Treatment Centre (co-ed)**
123 Franklyn Road, Kelowna
1-250-860-4001

Kinghaven Treatment Centre (men)
31250 King Road, Abbotsford
1-604-864-0039

**Maple Ridge
Treatment Centre (co-ed)**
22269 Callaghan Avenue, Maple Ridge
604-467-3471
Toll free: 1-877-678-6782 or 1-877-678-
MRTC
email: info@mrtc.bc.ca

Pacifica (co-ed)
1755 East 11th Avenue, Vancouver
604-872-5517

Path to Freedom (men)
19030 Highway #10, Surrey
604-576-6466

**Phoenix Drugs and Alcohol
Treatment Centre (men)**
13686 95A Avenue, Surrey
604-584-7166

RECOVERY HOUSES

Central City Lodge
415 West Pender Street, Vancouver
604-681-9111

Choices
695 Balmoral Street, Vancouver
604-325-6994

Cornerstone
10078 138 Street, Surrey
604-589-6060

Finally Free
9443-140 Street, Surrey
604-507-4244

Freedom House
13765 105 Avenue, Surrey
604-580-2783

Harbour Light
119 East Cordova Street, Vancouver
604-646-6800

Inner Visions Recovery
1937 Prairie Avenue, Port Coquitlam
604-468-2032

It's Up to You
(1st stage recovery house)
12991 100th Avenue, Surrey
604-580-1912

It's Up to You
(2nd stage recovery house)
1622 East 12th Avenue, Vancouver
604-254-5392

Lana House (men)
407 Kelly Street, New Westminster
604-524-3969

Last Door Recovery Society
328 8th Street, New Westminster
604-525-3896

Lifelines
12497 96th Avenue, Surrey
604-783-5170

Luke 15 House
11861 99th Avenue, Surrey
604-930-4346

New Day (men)
7533 143rd Street, Surrey
778-838-9927

Reflections (men)
8332 150th Street, Surrey
604-376-3457

Resurrection House
3237 Liverpool Street, Port Coquitlam
604-464-0475

Safe Haven
13574 79A Avenue, Surrey
604-572-6688

Shae Summit
9575 132A Street, Surrey
604-418-7296

Standing Strong
14128 Park Drive, Surrey
778-996-5249

Step by Step
12442 78A Avenue, Surrey
604-591-3153

Union Gospel Mission
616 East Cordova Street, Vancouver
604-253-3323

Wager Hills
8061 264th Street, Langley
604-856-9432

Welcome Home
6925 King George Avenue, Surrey
604-592-3004

Wellness House
1507 West 66th Avenue, Vancouver
604-267-1475

RESOURCES FOR PHYSICIANS AND ALLIED HEALTH CARE WORKERS

The College of Physicians and Surgeons of BC offers accredited courses and day workshops that enable licensed physicians to obtain the necessary certification to practice both Addiction Medicine and Mental Health. The basic requirement is the *Methadone 101* workshop offered biannually. Other courses are periodically scheduled that lead to certification by the Canadian Society of Addiction Medicine. The College website is: www.cpsbc.ca

REFERENCES

American Psychiatric Association. *The Diagnostic and Statistical Manual of Psychiatric Illness-IVR (DSM-IVR): Diagnosis, Etiology and Treatment.* Washington, DC: American Psychiatric Publishing, Inc., 2004.

Basch, Paul F. *Textbook of International Health*, New York: Oxford University Press, 1990.

Beattie, Melody. *The Language of Letting Go*, USA: Hazelden Foundation, 1990.

Carpenter, W.T. Jr, D.W. Heinricks and A.M.I. Wagman. "Deficit and nondeficit forms of schizophrenia: the concept," *American Journal of Psychiatry* 1988: 145: 578-583.

Cohen, B., J. Lipinski and R. Altesman. "Lecithin in the treatment of mania: double-blind placebo-controlled trials," *American Journal of Psychiatry* 1982: 139: 1162-64.

Dawkins, Richard. *The God Delusion.* New York: Mariner Books, 2006.

Doniger, Wendy. *The Hindus – An Alternative History.* New York: Penguin Press, 2009.

Epstein, M. *Thoughts Without a Thinker: Psychotherapy From A Buddhist Perspective.* New York: Basic Books, 1995.

Frawley, D. *Ayurveda and the Mind: The Healing of Consciousness.* Delhi: Motilal Banarsidass Publishers Private Ltd., 1997.

Green, Lawrence W. and Marshall W. Kreuter. *Health Promotion Planning – An Educational and Environmental Approach. Second Edition.* Mountain View, CA: Mayfield Publishing Co., 1991.

Kale, A. and S. Kale. *Tantra: The Secret Power of Sex.* Mumbai: Jaico Publishing House, 2002.

MacQueen, G.M., and L.T. Young and R.T. Joffe. "A review of psychosocial outcomes in patients with bipolar disorder," *Acta Psychiatr Scand.* 2001: 103: 163-170.

Manji Husseini K et al. "The underlying neurobiology of bipolar disorder," *World Psychiatry*, 2003 October 2 (3): 136-146.

Maté, Gabor. *Scattered Minds: A New Look at the Origins and Healing of Attention Deficit Disorder. First Edition.* Toronto: Vintage Canada, 2000.

Maté, Gabor. *In the Realm of Hungry Ghosts: Close Encounters with Addiction.* Toronto: Vintage Canada, 2009.

Melody, P. *Facing Codependence.* San Francisco: Harper Collins, 1989.

National Coalition on Dual Diagnosis (Canada). Dual diagnosis: Coping with mental health problems when you have a developmental disability. Position paper 2008. http://www.camh.net/Public_policy/Public_policy_papers/Position%20statement.pdf

Osho, R. *This Very Body the Buddha.* Mumbai: Jaico Publishing House, 1978.

Osho, R. *The First Principle: Talks on Zen.* Mumbai: Jaico Publishing House, 2006.

Osho, R. *From Sex to Superconsciousness.* New Delhi: Full Circle Publishing, 2006.

Pert, Candace. *Molecules of Emotion: Why you feel the way you feel.* New York: Scribner, 1997.

Robinson, David J. *The Personality Disorders Explained. Second Edition.* London, Ontario: Rapid Psychler Press, 2003.

Stoll, A., W. Severus, M. Freeman *et al.* "Omega-3 fatty acids in bipolar disorder: a preliminary double-blind placebo controlled trial," *Archives of General Psychiatry*, 1999: 56: 407-412.

Tacey, D. *Jung.* London: Granta Publications, 2006.

Whitfield, Charles L. *Boundaries and Relationships: Knowing, Protecting and Enjoying the Self.* Deerfield Beach, FL: Health Communications Inc., 1993.

Whitfield, Charles L. *Co-Dependence: Healing the Human Condition: The New Paradigm for Helping Professionals and People in Recovery.* Deerfield Beach, FL: Health Communications Inc., 1991.

Wilber, K. *Sex, Ecology, Spirituality.* Boston: Shambhala Publications, 1995.

Wilber, K. *A Brief History of Everything. Second Edition.* Boston: Shambhala Publications, 2000.

Brodbeck, S. *The Bhagavad Gita*. London: Penguin, 2003.

Burton, Sir R. and F.F. Arbuthonot. *Kamasutra of Vatsyayana*. Mumbai: Jaico Publishing House, 2002.

Campbell, Joseph with Bill Moyers. *The Power of Myth*. Mystic Fire Video: Parabola. New York. 1988.

Campbell, Joseph. *The Hero's Journey: Joseph Campbell On His Life and Work*. San Francisco: Harpercollins, 1990.

Campbell, Joseph. Transformations of Myth Through Time. New York: Harper Perennial Library, 1990.

Chopra, Deepak. *Ageless Body, Timeless Mind: The Quantum Alternative to Growing Old*. New York: Three Rivers Press, 1994.

Das, Lama Surya. *Awakening to The Sacred: Creating a Spiritual Life from Scratch*. New York: Broadway Books, 1999.

Feibleman, James K. *Understanding Oriental Philosophy. Revised Edition*. New York: Horizon Press, 1976.

Feuerstein, G. *Teachings of Yoga*. Boston: Shambhala, 1997.

Hawking, Stephen. *A Brief History of Time*. New York: Bantam Books, 1998.

Hawking, Stephen. *The Universe in a Nutshell*. New York: Bantam Books, 2001.

Iyengar, B.K.S. *Light on Yoga*. London: Harper Collins, 2001.

Krishnamurti, J. *Commentaries on Living. Third Edition*. New York: Harper, 1960.

Krishnamurti, J. *Fire in the Mind: Dialogues with J Krishnamurti*. New Delhi: Penguin Books, 1995.

Krishnamurti, J. *On Love and Loneliness*. San Francisco: Harper Collins Publishers, 1995.

Krishnamurti, J. *On Fear*. New York: Harper Collins Publishers, 1995.

Krishnamurti, J. *The Nature of the New Mind*. Chennai, India: Krishnamurti Foundation, 2001.

Krishnamurti, J. *The Mind of J. Krishnamurti*. Mumbai: Jaico Publishing House, 2007.

Lewis, C.S. *Mere Christianity*. New York: Macmillan Publishing Co., 1960.

Maharaj, Sri Nisargadatta. *I Am That: Selected Talks*. Durham, CA: Acorn Press, 1973.

Merton, Thomas. *The Ascent to Truth*. Orlando, FL : Harcourt, Brace and Co., 1981.

Merton, Thomas. *Mystics and Zen Masters*. New York: Farrar, Strauss and Girous, 1967.

Ramacharaka, Y. *Lessons in Gnani Yoga*. Chicago, IL: The Yogi Publication Society, 1934.

Ramacharaka, Y. *Advanced Course in Yogi Philosophy and Oriental Occultism*. Varanasi: Pilgrims Publishing, 2008.

Rumi, J. A. *Spiritual Treasury*. Oxford: Oneworld Publications, 2000.

Satchidananda, Sri Swami. *The Yoga Sutras of Patanjali: Translation and Commentary*. USA: Integral Yoga Publications, 1990.

Shah, Idries. *The Way of the Sufi*. Suffolk, UK: Penguin Books, 1974.

Shumsky, Susan G. *Exploring Chakras: Awaken Your Untapped Energy. First Indian Edition*. New Delhi: New Page Books, 2006.

Sivaraman, K. *Hindu Spirituality: Vedas Through Vedanta*. Delhi: Motilal Banarsidass Publishers Private Ltd., 1989.

Tagore, Rabindranath. *Selected Poems*. New Delhi: Oxford University Press, 2004.

Tolle, Eckhart. *The Power of Now*. Novato, CA: New World Library, 1999.

Tolle, Eckhart. *A New Earth: Awakening to Your Life's Purpose*. London: Penguin Books, 2005.

Watts, Alan W. *The Way of Zen*. New York: Vintage Books, 1957.

Watts, Alan W. *The Wisdom of Insecurity: A Message for an Age of Anxiety*. New York: Vintage Books, 1960.

Watts, Alan W. *The Essential Alan Watts*. Berkeley, CA: Celestial Arts, 1977.

Watts, Alan W. *Still the Mind: An Introduction to Meditation*. Novato, CA: New World Library, 2000.

Watts, Alan W. *Out of Your Mind*. Boulder, CO: Sounds True, 2004.

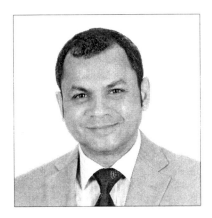

Dr. Robert Bernard Pereira received his Bachelor of Science degree in Biochemistry from the University of British Columbia in 1986 and went on to complete his medical degree at UBC in 1990. A certificant of the Canadian College of Family Physicians (CCFP), he has completed two years of postgraduate medical training in the Department of Health Care and Epidemiology at UBC, working towards a Master of Health Science degree (MHSc).

Dr. Pereira is currently pursuing accreditation with both the American Board and Canadian Society of Addiction Medicine (ABAM and CSAM). He holds licenses to prescribe methadone to treat opiate addiction and chronic pain and is one of the few physicians in BC who is licensed to prescribe Suboxone® for the treatment of opiate addiction.

Dr. Pereira has recently completed a mentorship program at the Liver and Intestinal Research Centre (LAIR) in Vancouver under the pupilage of Dr. Frank H. Anderson. Dr. Pereira will soon be undertaking a mentorship program in

HIV-coinfection under the pupilage of internationally renowned infectious disease specialist Dr. John Farley in Vancouver, BC.

Dr. Pereira is married and lives in Ladner, BC. He divides his time between a busy practice in family medicine in Surrey and an affiliated addiction and mental health practice in Surrey and downtown Vancouver.

When not working, writing or speaking, Dr. Pereira enjoys researching alternative forms of medicine, in particular psychospiritual applications, and traveling. He collects rare Indian artifacts related to the gods and myths of India.

CONTACT INFORMATION

FOR DR. ROBERT B. PEREIRA

website: www.dualdiagnosis.ca

email: info@dualdiagnosis.ca

CPSIA information can be obtained at www.ICGtesting.com
Printed in the USA
LVOW130705251011

251897LV00003B/1/P